Don't Call Me Home

Don't Call Me Home

A Memoir

Alexandra Auder

VIKING

VIKING
An imprint of Penguin Random House LLC
penguinrandomhouse.com

LIBRARY OF CONGRESS CATALOGING-IN-PUBLICATION DATA
Names: Auder, Alexandra, author.
Title: Don't call me home : a memoir / Alexandra Auder.
Description: New York : Viking, 2023.
Identifiers: LCCN 2022043598 (print) | LCCN 2022043599 (ebook) |
ISBN 9780593299951 (hardcover) | ISBN 9780593299968 (ebook)
Subjects: LCSH: Auder, Alexandra. | Viva, 1938—Family. |
Yoga teachers—United States—Biography. |
Actors—United States—Biography. |
Children of celebrities—United States—Biography.
Classification: LCC RA781.67 A83 2023 (print) |
LCC RA781.67 (ebook) | DDC 613.7/046092 [B]—dc23/eng/20221201
LC record available at https://lccn.loc.gov/2022043598
LC ebook record available at https://lccn.loc.gov/2022043599

Printed in the United States of America
1st Printing

Designed by Amanda Dewey

Some names and identifying characteristics have been
changed to protect the privacy of the individuals involved.

For Mom,
thanks for paving the way

"Viva was there with her daughter Alexandra who was sucking her thumb. Seeing Alexandra was sad—a big rug-rat hanging off Viva—she'll probably turn out a mess. Viva will do everything the opposite that her parents did and it'll be just as bad."

—ANDY WARHOL, *The Andy Warhol Diaries*

CONTENTS

Part 3. THE OUTER WORLD: *1986–1989*

Now

I grab a steak knife from the kitchen and march upstairs. As I pass Nick, my husband, he shoots me a reprimanding look. I roll my eyes at him. But we both know what I am capable of.

Remember to be nice, she has only been here for a day!

There she is, ensconced in my seven-year-old son Miko's bed, wrapped in his *Star Wars* sheets, her flannel nightgown open at her chest. Her chest marked with the harbingers of what will come for me—no, what has come for me: liver spots.

It's the same chest the full-of-shit doctor tossed me on, the same chest I once wanted to live inside of, the same chest I rested my cheek against as a child, the same chest I longed for when she was away, and the same chest I am now imagining plunging this knife into.

Why would I want to stab a beautiful but weakened eighty-year-old grandmother with a healthy head of hair who is recovering from a journey across the country?

"I think I'm dying," she says, as I approach her.

She is at my house for Christmas, convalescing. Convalescing, like talking on the phone, is her sport.

"Hand me the pills," I demand.

Now she meekly hands over one of the open bottles filled with tiny pills.

"I'm dying," she repeats, as if I hadn't heard the first time. This means nothing to me; it's birdsong.

I let one pill fall into my hand and place it on a book. I rest the edge of the knife against the sliver of the dividing line on the pill, and cup the knife and pill with one hand while applying pressure with the other, suggesting with my false confidence that only a moron needs a pill cutter. Whatever a pill cutter is. I hadn't known they existed until I deciphered the text she sent me earlier:

Pill Cutter

Mexican Coke

Flan

Gaffer Tape

"Your eyes are still so good. You don't need glasses? Wow, honey! I can't even see the pill . . ."

She is leaning in, trying to peer under my hands to make sure I've split the pill correctly.

I'm forty-seven, so I do actually need reading glasses, but I was too proud to grab them before the procedure; still there's the impulse to seize upon my mother's weaknesses, hold them over her head and flaunt my strengths, just as my fifteen-year-old, Lui, flaunts her exquisite youth, while Miko obsesses over the aging process, examining the skin on my hands while we cuddle in bed and asking if I'll be wrinkled like Grandma by the time he gets to college, or if I'll even still be alive.

I could die tomorrow, I'm tempted to say.

I feel the pill crisply snap into two clean pieces.

Relief.

Anyway, what could a weak older woman with diarrhea do to me if I had accidentally crushed one of her last remaining migraine pills? If she had peered under my hand and seen white powder rather than two tiny white half-moons?

"I can't be*lieve* you were able to do that without a pill cutter!" she squeals with childish delight. And then, with the tiny voice of a consumption victim begging for her cure, the question I knew would come: "Did you get me a Mexican Coke?"

"They didn't have it," I mumble.

She hates when I mumble. The truth is I am sure "they" had it—the Mexican take-out place a few blocks away—but I was too annoyed to make an extra stop—and I'm hoping she will assume that I'm referring to the CVS.

"Mi Puebla didn't have it?!" she asks incredulously.

Shit. She remembers. Everywhere we have ever lived she has clocked where the Mexican Coke is sold.

I look around the room. She has eviscerated a suitcase meant for one week of living away from home—Palm Springs—but which could actually sustain two or three humans and one animal for six to eight months. There are at least five half-full glasses of various liquids. An open box of saltines. A yogurt-encrusted spoon sitting in a pool of coagulated fat from a chunk of steak I don't remember any of us cooking. Used tissues spread about the room like blossoms on lawns at the end of spring. A dozen bottles of pills. An open Vaseline jar and paint-splattered brown Birkenstocks. Large scissors sitting open on the floor, great for Miko to step on. A newspaper from Palm Springs, rubber gloves, and pills scattered around the floor that one or both of us have accidentally crushed with our feet, which might be why she accidentally took a lorazepam instead of an Ativan.

And the red enema bag.

Hi there, old friend.

I sit on Miko's bed trying to decide if I should tackle the mess. Or let her wallow in it? I have intentionally tried to shore myself up against the tidal push to complain. I hold my not complaining over my mother's head. But what has that done for me? Left me belly-up on the shore of beached martyrs, that's what.

This is the first time she bought a return ticket home. I can do this for ten days.

Her feet are swishing against each other under the covers. When I do this, Lui says I have to get away from her.

My mother takes my hand into hers. "Oh, honey, it's hell getting old, total hell."

We have the same thumbs. They're called murderer's thumbs. Our thumbs are shorter than normal thumbs, narrow at the base and bulbous at the top. Lui has one of our thumbs and one of Nick's, which is a normal thumb. My mother lets her thumbnails grow long enough to clear the bulbous fleshy tips, which I find disturbing. The actual nail bed on a murderer's thumb is a miniature rectangle. One horizontal swipe of a nail polish brush turned on its side can fill it in, especially if you bite these nails, which Lui and I do. My mother can't stand nail-biting. She can't stand any bodily picking that other people do. She, of course, picks freely.

Now she raises her arm up as if to whack my hand away from my mouth like she did when I was a kid, but I jerk away from her before she has a chance to make contact. She senses this could be a dangerous thing to do. I've got the upper hand sizewise and strengthwise.

"Lots of chemtrails today," she says, looking out the window, breaking the silence.

"It's condensation."

"OK, honey, believe what you want to believe."

She loves Proust but doesn't believe we landed on the moon; she understands string theory but thinks 9/11 was an inside job.

Be nice, be nice, be nice, I chant to myself.

I was lucky to have my bare newborn skin connect with her skin, to be generously nursed for years, my body cuddled, my imagination nurtured . . . so why is it that rather than wanting to thank my mother by anointing her crepey-thin skin, rather than wanting to hold her in my arms and assuage her fear of sickness and death, rather than wanting to help usher her soul back to the universal womb . . . I want to smother her?

I want to pry her eyelids open and force her to reckon with "the truth"—ha!—and relish the moment when her voice, raspy with awe, whispers: *the horror, the horror.*

Part 1

PLACE TO PLACE

1971–1980

Chapter 1

The Beginning

Viva walks out of the elevators of the Chelsea Hotel wearing a hooded, ankle-length djellaba over her huge belly. She collapses into a sudden heap and moans dramatically, fabric billowing around her on the bright red rug.

I know the lobby rug is red because it is as close as skin to me: I grew up crawling, then walking, then roller-skating, then slinking around and hiding in the halls of this hotel. But this particular memory is in black and white. It's not a real memory—I wasn't born yet, but I'm about to be.

My earliest memories have been permanently hijacked by my father's video camera.

At this point in our lives, the camera is a classic Sony Portapak—a hulking object that weighs a ton—but his exciting new version of film makes memory light on its toes, and it obsesses my father, Michel.

Growing up, as the video cameras get smaller and smaller, I will watch my life come into being, on loop, on a little black-and-white video monitor, and these images will bleed into my actual memories and make it hard to tell the difference between the two.

I will say, "I want to see Emma born!" but here, again, the truth has been hijacked. When I say Emma, I mean *me*. That's because in 1973, my mom will write a book called *The Baby*, in which she will use Michel's video stills as illustrations and which they will call a video novel—a protoversion of today's graphic novel. *The Baby* will be about the birth of Emma, who is really me, and Emma's life with Frederique, who is really Michel. Critics will call our lives a funnier, more honest, and (notably) *female* version of Kerouac's *On the Road*. "An extraordinary verbal videotape of a life in the process of being lived," Joan Didion will say. "Enchanting, or maybe enchanted." On the street in Paris, Simone de Beauvoir, somewhat cryptically, will tell my mother that she thinks her transcription style of tape recordings will be the future of fiction writing.

For any of this to happen—to matter—the camera will always be recording, the moment of my mother's water breaking just another in a string of documented moments between brushing her teeth and arguing with the cops.

This is a video memory.

She is now sprawled out on the floor of the lobby, propping herself up with one arm, the djellaba forming a tent around her body, her slender feet sticking out. She groans, rocking back and forth and rhythmically wiggling her feet together. (The foot thing, which I will inherit, is a habit that will eventually drive me crazy, and will eventually drive my daughter, Lui, crazy.)

"Don't worry, don't worry. Breez, *breeeez*," my father croons in his French accent from behind the camera. He's not lending a hand, but he's making a good effort to sound concerned. He is long-haired and probably wearing his uniform—green velvet tight pants, a threadbare striped cowboy shirt, and lots of silver rings and brace-lets. Jerry, the man behind the desk, also keeps his distance. As my mother makes animal noises, he stays behind the desk, where he will remain until I leave for college.

"It's gonna be a girl!" Jerry yells out like a sports announcer.

"I don't know," my mother responds wearily.

"*Breeeez!*" my father repeats.

My father's voice is the one I will come to know well, the voice he uses when he's filming. It's distracted—like when you are watching television and someone asks you a question and you answer without tearing your eyes from the screen. But in my father's case, this is a voice he uses often around living, breathing people—people, like my mother, giving birth.

Now they are walking out of the lobby, pushing open the heavy glass doors, stepping onto Twenty-third Street between Seventh and Eighth Avenues. They stand, perfectly framed, under the red and white striped Chelsea awning, wedding cake figures in bell bottoms and harem robes.

"What you think it's going to be—girl or boy?" my father asks the bellman, who is waving down a cab.

"A girl! I want a girl!" the bellman says in a Spanish accent.

The whole Chelsea has an opinion.

MY MOTHER HAD tried to abort me. But she missed the appointment, she says, because a friend of my father's got her too stoned.

She had met my father, Michel, on the streets of Paris, just after she'd filmed the sex scene in Warhol's *Blue Movie* that would make her both superstar and criminal. She and Michel made off for Rome (both draped in ruffled silk shirts, jewel-toned velvet blazers, capes, beaded necklaces, and chunky silver bracelets) to make their own movie, ironically titled *Keeping Busy*, and then to Hollywood, so my mother could star in Agnès Varda's *Lions Love* in order to make enough money to finish the movie in Rome.

In retelling these stories, Viva always blames my father for the way the narrative unfolded. He was too reckless, or too high, or too much of a "gigolo," or too obsessed with his videotaping—or all of it at the same time.

During a dinner party at Jane Fonda and Roger Vadim's house in Hollywood, my father "forced" my mother to smoke too much hash, and she then became paranoid about Michel kissing Sharon Tate in the library. (Or maybe, as Michel recalls, it was Barbarella in the kitchen.) Regardless, he was kissing some other beautiful woman, and before anyone knew it, Jane Fonda was telling my mother to "go marry him in Vegas," and so off they went.

The marriage, my mother says, was only because Fonda suggested it. My mother used the Fonda name to book a hotel and wore black satin pajamas to the altar. My father filmed the whole thing, of course, but the film was ruined or lost, which, my mother says, was all my father's fault.

So she never had the abortion; instead, my mother filmed a few scenes with Kris Kristofferson in the movie *Cisco Pike*. In one scene she was naked and pregnant with me, lounging on a bed as Merna, a socialite groupie. During the scene, I was waiting to be born.

WE ARE IN the delivery room. Those irritating ankles are *swish, swish, swish*ing together on the crisp hospital sheets. My mother is lying in a fetal position, groaning and rocking. She has short curly hair like a cherub's and her head is thrown back. She's letting out primitive sounds that rise slowly in pitch and seem to reverberate around the bare hospital walls. There is heavy, rhythmic breathing coming from deep within her body.

Later, while I watch this video, I will sync my own breath in time with hers, unintentionally trying to get closer to the birth experience. Much later, as I lay in bed next to her, I will again quietly sync my breath with hers in order to avoid inhaling any of her exhaled breath, as though her breath is an entity that could invade my body and disrupt my inner world.

Suddenly, she releases a big scream, and then there it is: her pussy, looking nothing like one. It's really huge and bulbous, as big as a bald man's head with a ridiculous curly toupee sitting on top.

"It's coming!" the doctor says, and then as if conjured, the top of my head appears through the huge slit, accompanied by an agonized wail. The head looks like an exposed brain, all wrinkled and gray.

Tight close-up of the pussy here. (My father's creative direction.)

As an adult, when I watch this moment with friends, screen trained on my mother's vagina, I say, "Look at the head coming out!"—as though the baby is Emma, not me. I intentionally try to embody myself as a newborn, but it's impossible to do while watching oneself on a screen.

Meanwhile, the doctor makes an incision toward the perineum (a decision my mother will audibly lament every time we watch it). She yelps just as the labial skin bursts open on the screen, a flower blooming on time-lapse film. The blue head pops out of the vagina and the bloody slit below it, and the doctor clamps the umbilical cord, which is wrapped tightly around the baby's neck, and then cuts it; as he does so, he wipes the baby's (my) squished-up face with his hand and squeezes the (my) head, rotating it around the opening of the vagina as though he is trying to break this baby's (my) neck. He is aggressive, always too aggressive. (They hired this particular one, my father tells me later, because he was the only one who would let them film the birth. "He was full of shit," my mother always says.)

After another wipe of the face, it's me. I let out a wail and my body seems to slip out easily, almost gracefully.

My father, laughing, says off-screen, "Sounds like a boy!"

The full-of-shit doctor catches my back with one hand, my bottom with the other; my body is face up now, fitting nicely into his palms, my legs fall open, frog-like, and my swollen vagina appears. I am, indeed, a girl.

"Ah, Miss Auder," the doctor says, holding me, but looking between my mother's legs. "Do you want it medium or snug?" he asks her.

"Michel," my mother says wryly, "how do you want my cunt?"

The doctor tosses me onto my mother's chest like a little rubber doll, and there, for the first time in the outside world, I meet my true love face-to-face.

Chapter 2

Family Diaries

The first five years of my life are all video memories: scenes and moments my father captured, and edited, and replayed for me over the years.

THE CHELSEA HOTEL.

My father films as my mother emerges from the bathtub, looking into the video camera.

"I'm sick of being a star. It's like being a slave. This is my last performance," she complains.

She moves toward the bed, naked, and dripping wet with that peculiar slow-motion walk, like a drunkard. Her breasts are like swollen torpedoes, jigging as she approaches me. I'm lying on my back on the bed, kicking my legs, my bald head turned toward her, my mouth gaping, apparently rapt by her breasts.

Now she lounges on the bed, me next to her, a white towel wrapped like a turban around her head. I am exploring the shadows, ridges, and plays of light on her face while I nurse and she talks to the camera. The cloudy, sweet milk seems to melt my limbs.

A topless woman is also sprawled out here in our bedroom in the hotel—my godmother, Brigid Berlin, another Warhol actress. She has rolls of flesh and fat and drones on and on in the same hypnotic way as my mother. A continuous monologue flows from both women, like they are the stars of the world's longest opera. My mother's palm covers the skin on my back, as if she's sending silent love notes into my body while she laughs at something Brigid is saying.

My father continues to film as Brigid attaches a recording device to the phone—a little black rubber suction cup. Andy Warhol's voice emerges from the other end of the line.

"Andy—why haven't you called to find out about Alexandra?" Brigid drones, deadpan. "She's so beautiful. And why haven't you called Viva?"

"Oh, I haven't had time—I just got back. Is the baby good-looking?"

"Wonderful. Here, talk to Viva now."

Brigid hands my mother the phone.

"Well, Andy, I was going to make you the baby's godfather, but since you *still* haven't come to see us . . . I don't know . . . ," my mother says coyly, smiling at Brigid and the camera, clearly loving the fact that Andy hadn't known she was in the room when he was talking to Brigid.

"Everybody says you were just great on the television," he says.

"Oh yeah?"

"Yes, everyone loved you. They said you were fabulous. Are you going to any other shows soon? They would boost your book sales . . ."

"Well, they want me to do *Cavett* again tomorrow, but I'm just too exhausted."

"It would be good—"

"Andy, I'm not a *superhuman*. I can't have a baby and then rush right off to television a few days after—"

"Well, take the baby with you."

"The baby could go without me—sure, the baby will be fine—I'm the one . . . It was two hours of *excruciating pain*!"

"Are you taking a lot of vitamins?"

"I really think the pain was worse than the pain of your shooting."

"I'm sure it was terrible . . ."

"Can't they put something down there so that the pain won't hurt?"

"No matter what they give you, you still feel it—having the baby born wasn't painful . . . The baby coming out wasn't painful, it was . . . I thought my pain was just like the crucifixion—how did you feel?"

"Um . . . mine was so different . . . it was just hot . . . it was so weird . . . it was really sort of weird . . ."

"Well, you had drugs afterward, didn't you?"

"I can't remember . . . You know who I saw tonight? You're both from *Midnight Cowboy* . . . He really looks good . . . gee, I don't think anything ever really happened to him . . . he tried so hard . . . isn't that funny?"

"He who is first shall be last and he who is last shall be first."

"Uh-huh . . ."

"He who tries gets no place . . ."

"Uh-huh . . ."

"Christ."

LONDON.

My father films the hotel restaurant, empty except for a long table seating about twelve English businessmen. They won't seat us because I'm nursing.

Michel yells: *"We want a menu!"*

His voice behind the camera sounds irritated, hollowed by adrenaline.

My mother stands in front of the table of Englishmen and orates to them: "I am sure one of you gentlemen must have one child among you—surely you're not that uptight that you can't even *conceive a child*!"

They continue eating without looking up.

The hotel manager approaches us with his hands out toward the camera. My father says, *"Don't touch it, don't come near me, it iz off . . . I will punch you . . ."* He laughs a little when he says this.

The maître'd tries to pry the camera from Michel and there is a big scuffle. Suddenly, lots of hands are jabbing and poking around my head. My father yells: *"We need a police officer!"*

The next day my father videotapes the covers of the London *Sun* and the New York *Daily News*: "Warhol Actress Arrested for Indecency in London Hotel."

MOROCCO.

My father films as I take my first wobbly steps in a nomad's cave, through a cloud of hash smoke, my feet just clearing the hem of my little djellaba. Outside, thousands of little blackbirds fly in and out of oblong patterns against the pale sky.

My father films my mother and me on our jerky camel ride. Nearby, kids are playing in the wind-whipped sand with material wrapped around their heads.

My father films as I watch my mother applying black liquid eyeliner and flaring her nostrils in the mirror. When she talks, she holds up a hand like saints do in old paintings—her arm bent at the elbow, palm facing outward, as though she is making a benevolent offering.

I have short curly hair and a heart-shaped mouth. I'm absorbed by watching her put on her makeup and talk; I look sleepy, like someone is tickling my back.

My mother says she is worried about my diarrhea.

The Chelsea Hotel.

My father films our trashed kitchen after he and my mother fight. I'm in a sink full of sudsy water. The black-and-white linoleum squares are littered with broken plates and spilled garbage.

My father films me toddling through the marble halls of the Chelsea with a curly-haired girl I call Padamimi; we are smiling, laughing, and we both take a nip of milk from her mother's nipple.

My father films me wandering barefoot along the sidewalk of Twenty-third Street. I've got fuller hair now with curls to my shoulders. The striped Chelsea awning is in front of us. I pass beautiful piles of black-and-white garbage; my "friend," a bum who lived under the stoop next to the toy store; and the offtrack betting shop where the sad men loiter. We pass the impossibly narrow comic store and the El Quijote. Above us, stacked ten stories high, are the little Chelsea balconies with their curlicue-shaped wrought iron railings.

Topanga.

My father films me outside our lopsided house, one that seems to teeter over the edge of a cliff. I am climbing up dusty piles of canyon dirt wearing polyester flared pants and a turtleneck with a scalloped hem. Fat muddy cheeks and ratty hair. I am having a *fuck you* screaming match with a boy pointing a toy gun at me.

My father films me as I pile up my stuffed animals—a stack of three or four—and hump them, with abandon, until I get the good tingly feeling that I have recently discovered.

My mother brings me to a tall man in orange robes named Muktananda, who tells me that this thing I do to get the good tingly feeling is fine—"it's like rubbing your tummy," he says.

My mother films me now, and here is a rare sighting of my father. He sings me the "ko ko nuts" song, and dances with a white towel wrapped around his narrow waist, his long hair trailing down his bare back.

My father films me as I tell the camera, "I have to shit." I say it to make my cousin Steve laugh. I love the way words like *Valium* and *fucker* and *shit* sound when I say them to the camera, and I like watching them later with Steve. He is not allowed to curse. His mother, my aunt Barb, recently told me that I shouldn't say *I love you* so often either.

My father films me watching myself on the videos he has already made—the videos from New York, London, Morocco. It makes me nostalgic for the Chelsea.

———

AND THEN THE VIDEO memories end. My real memories begin.

I MUST HAVE BEEN close to five when I found my parents on a mattress on the floor, breathing heavily, like dogs playing, growling, baring their teeth. My mother whimpered while my father straddled her, forcing something into her mouth—a pill maybe?

Soon after this, it seemed, a familiar man sat on a chair across from us. We were all waiting for something—some big decision to just happen. My father was standing in the open doorway to the outside. He was out of breath and agitated. My mother seemed calm.

Are you coming or not? my father asked me. He was looking at me. *If you don't come with me now, you'll never see me again.*

He didn't laugh.

I was very still, maybe lead in my blood. *How long will they wait for my answer? One hundred thousand years?* I wanted to *not* go with him, to stay with my mother, but make it so that he didn't know that I was not going with him. I stilled myself. First, the peripheral edges of my body, then the inside, slowly folding it up like an accordion closing. Maybe I was invisible, but I felt more solid, like petrified wood. I waited for them to realize I was unreachable; I was resting, deep, deep inside, hidden by the calcified layers.

I don't know how long they waited.

Later, Viva and Michel stopped the car and abandoned our dogs, Tupi and Lapa, on the side of a dusty canyon road, strips of eucalyptus bark in the gutter, and drove away from Topanga Canyon. We may have driven away together, as a family unit, but I remember it as the split.

We left Michel—or he left us—and my mother and I fused.

Chapter 3

On the Road

After the split, my mother and I roamed. We roamed like two nomads on the lam, in a broken-down car, with no heat and a cat we had picked up somewhere along the way, climbing the Rockies, winding through tiny roads of aspen, traversing the hot canyons of LA, briefly settling here and there.

I'd watch her in profile from the passenger seat. Commanding nose, a vigilant large blue eye, a high cheekbone held in place by smooth alabaster skin, and a frizzy halo of strawberry blond hair. The same profile on the jacket of her first book, *Superstar*, with the one eye on the spine of the book. "Vivah Supahstahhhh!" I often blurted out because I liked the way it sounded. "I luv ya, Vivah Supahstahhhh!"

We would stop on the side of the highway so I could rub my mother's frozen feet. She would take off her shoes, and I'd pull off her thick wool socks edged by a red stripe and hold her slender feet in my lap, rubbing them back to life.

"I was a foot model," she told me.

I was impressed.

We listened to opera on the radio. I wanted to be an opera singer, though I had no musical talent at all, but I would sing along anyhow, making my voice waver.

I also had a pretty good southern accent that I used to sing country style and she *loved* that. I thought if I didn't make it as an opera star I'd try country. Making up the lyrics as we drove, I sang about the images as they passed us, folk music style, sprinkling the phrases with a few rhyming obscenities. "There's a cooow in a field, seeeee the milk in their tiiits? Oh, sure it's true, sweet baby, that one fine daaay . . . they'll have to take some shiiits!"

On the road, my mother ate the fried clam sandwiches from Howard Johnson's, claiming they were the best there. Sometimes she ate her sandwich in the car with her favorite milkshake, a black and white malted.

People who didn't know what she knew were either morons or needed her mentoring. If the ice-cream parlor kid didn't know what a black and white was, she would walk him through it: "You don't have them? Of course you do, honey," she would say. "It's just vanilla ice cream with chocolate *syrup* and malt—you've got malt, don't you? Here, let me see." Suddenly, she'd be behind the counter in the kitchen. "Whew! It's filthy back here . . ."

She also liked flan, Coke, and sherbet, which she pronounced "sher-*bit*." When she was sick, those things were her medicine. If she had a headache, she would say, "I've got to stop and get a Coke, honey." Or, if she had diarrhea, she would say: "I've got to get some flan and rest."

When she got too tired to drive, she would pull up to a motel lot, and I would duck down in the car and steal glances of her through the office window and admire her beauty. My love for her burned the inside of my chest.

After she got the key, she would march back to the car, drive away from the office, park in front of the room, open the door, come back and whisper, "Hurry, take the cat and run in!"

Inside we would lie in a single motel bed together while I watched the little black-and-white television mounted on the ceiling, and she worried about things. I listened to her worries while I luxuriated in her smell—the smell that made me go heavy in her arms and slide my thumb into my mouth.

AT ONE POINT during the roam, we briefly settled in a spacious house in Miami, where she was writing a screenplay.

While we were there, she finally let me go to *Jaws*, a movie I had become obsessed with when I saw the ads. After I'd seen it, though, when I had to go to the bathroom, I made her come with me. I needed her to stay while I was on the toilet—just in case the nose of a shark came exploding out.

Each time I went to the bathroom, I quizzed her in order to distract her from the fact that I was scared; otherwise she would say she *never* should have let me see that movie.

I tried to sound casual. With her voice in the room I could relax my bladder.

I loved her voice. I always asked her the same questions. There was a special wrapping around each answer, like each contained a secret code and only she—out of all the moms in the universe— knew the real meaning. I took mental notes.

"What's your favorite color?"

"Magenta."

"What's your favorite food?"

"Pickled herrings. Or blintzes with sour cream and caviar."

"What's your favorite cartoon?"

"*Betty Boop.*"

I knew all the answers already, but I acted like I was hearing them for the first time.

"Favorite movie?"

"*Gone With the Wind.*"

"I love ya so much I could die!" I sang in a raspy voice that I used to imitate Rod Stewart. Then, after a pause, I tentatively asked: "Can sharks get into pools?"

"Oh my God, I *never* should have let you see that movie!!"

IN MEMPHIS WE STOPPED at an auto body shop where some greasy guys tried to fix our car. We had begun slowly rolling through red lights because if we actually had to come to a stop, we couldn't get the car started again.

"Those are the stupidest men I have ever seen in my entire life," she said afterward. "God, how I hate men. Remind me never to get involved with any man ever again."

I'll try, I thought.

A couple of times she had what I guess you would call lovers. I would have called them fucking assholes. Each dalliance was a stab in the heart. When she was interested in a man, her glistening flushed face and toothy smile were a betrayal as deep as any lover had ever felt. There were not many, but even so, I was gobsmacked every time it seemed that I wasn't enough for her. The fact that she wanted to spend time with someone other than me—and maybe even use that time to have *sex*—made her seem temporarily vulgar and ordinary.

But there was one I liked.

Bill Eggleston was married, a tall southern charmer, the drunk oracle of modern color photography, with a tousled swoosh of hair like a brushstroke of black ink on the top of his head. When he drank, his bow tie came unraveled, his face drooped over its own sharp, chiseled bones, and his black ink hair dripped down his temple.

I thought of him as her first boyfriend.

Bill, Viva, and I stayed in motels, surrounded by flat land and open space, under huge cobalt skies, with pools at their center. I'd stretch out on the plastic recliners by the pool and sunbathe with my clothes on while taking pictures of the sky with the Nikon camera Bill had given me to try to capture the light the way he had been teaching me.

Inside, on the dingy bedspreads, my mother was probably making love to him, which I loathed the thought of, but I would bear it and let it happen because I liked him.

The light, Bill had said to me, and I repeated to myself, *It's all in the light.*

BILL LEFT US in West Hollywood, in a single-story flat-roofed house next to a red poinsettia bush under a cloudless blue sky. My mother sat on the bare wood floor, sobbing. Her despair frightened me. I hugged her and wondered if he probably had to go back to his wife, Rosa ("Rowzah"), in Memphis, Tennessee, or maybe he drank too much and my mother had had enough.

We settled for a time in that lonely house. Maybe because we had paused our search for the next exciting thing, something had shifted. I began to dread her death and feared being left by her. On the rare occasions she would leave me with a sitter, I would go into her closet and bury my face in her magenta cotton dress, the one with a floral pattern. I would sniff it like a drug and try to forget everything until she got home.

When she did, I curled up in her lap like a baby, pressed my cheek against her bony freckled chest, drank in her smell, and listened to the beat of her heart.

She looked down at me when I moaned aloud.

"I don't want you to die," I said.

"Don't think about it, honey," she said, caressing my head.

"There are only two people I love more than you," I said.

"Who are they?"

She knew the answer, but I couldn't bear even the few seconds it took to deliver the punch line: "Nobody and nobody."

"Oh!" she howled. "You are *sooo* funny!"

"I love ya so much I could die!"

MY MOTHER BOUGHT me a red-eyed, white-furred rabbit. Maybe it was a consolation gift for an impending eye operation I was to have to correct my crossed eyes. I loved it, even though it would hide in the closet and bite me when I tried to pet it. But the rabbit soon escaped under the fence and disappeared in West Hollywood. That's when I began to worry even more that my mother would also disappear.

One afternoon I was convinced that it had actually happened. When I returned home from the school bus, I found our house empty. I stood out on our flat-white sidewalk under the violent blue sky and sobbed, letting the spit and tears drip everywhere. Our neighbor was rummaging through his trash. He stared at me, imitating my crying with a whiny nasal voice—*Wah, Wah, Wah.* I had always suspected he might have killed our rabbit, and right then, I imagined he must have had something to do with my mother's disappearance. At best, I suspected he was a sadist like my mother's friend from the Warhol days, Paul Morrissey. Paul would dangle candy above my head and yank it away just as I was about to grab it. He would taunt me with his nasal voice and tell me I was going to be taken away to a juvenile delinquent home.

Wah, Wah, Wah, Paul would say.

"Oh, ignore him, honey, he's a sadist," my mother would remind me. I thought a sadist was someone who didn't understand that I was my mother's equal, an intellectual extension of her. There were other sadists like Paul, other men who encouraged my mother to leave me at home, who spoke only to her, who avoided eye contact with me.

When the rabbit-slaughtering neighbor pulled out the butcher knife, I heard my mother's voice in my head: *Call the cops!* I did, but when they arrived, they appeared confused, unhelpful. They looked through our closets. They even looked for her in a shoebox.

"Drugs," she said later, while hugging me tight. "They were looking for drugs, the bastards." She had simply been at her sister Barb's house and had lost track of the time. "They probably thought that since I was a Warhol star I was a drug addict, the idiots."

I shook my head in acknowledgment.

"Viva *Superstar,*" I said.

"Ha," she said. "You are so smart."

I DON'T REMEMBER my father being around at all until after I got the eye operation.

I woke up with a patch over one eye and saw him standing at the foot of my moving bed holding a small tiger with a hard body covered in felt skin.

I realized I must have gone through something more dangerous than I had imagined, something serious enough to bring my father to the hospital.

The next time I saw him we were in a loft in Tribeca, and there was some sort of exchange meant to happen—me from him to my mother or from my mother to him. All I could feel was the stringy tension in the air. He was distant but trying to act relaxed and easy. My mother was suspicious, on guard. All of a sudden, like in a cowboy movie when the new guy in town enters the saloon and everyone has drawn their guns, my parents were chasing each other around the glass coffee table.

At first I thought it was a game, like tag. And then, I'm not sure how, it turned to fury. My mother was screaming things at Michel, mean things that I felt guilty about her saying. He was a *good-for-nothing dope addict*, he didn't care about me. I worried they would fall through the glass coffee table, bloody shards slicing their skin, puncturing their eyeballs.

My mother called the police.

My father laughed.

They approached the top of the hall stairs, struggling physically with each other. From behind, my father's frame looked like a giant shadow puppet on a white wall. He lifted my mother up, his hands on her waist, her frizzy hair sticking out from all sides. She looked slight between his hands, slight and sharp and taut, like the toy tiger he'd given me.

As her body seemed to hover above the stairwell, I ran into a bedroom and hid my head under a pillow and began to descend into the inner realms. Down, down, down I went, heart slowing, into the center of the petrified tree. A few moments later I felt the bed slump. I was under the calcified layers, but I could still hear his muffled voice.

"Don't worry," he said, out of breath. He was trying to sound relaxed, but I could feel his body trembling. "Your mozer iz not dead. Go ahead, go to her."

She was down on the sidewalk, hair standing on end, gesturing wildly to the cops, listing all the crimes my father had ever committed: *marijuana, using heroin, drug dealing, crashing and abandoning rental cars, stealing Christmas presents from Toys "R" Us!* This last thing on the list finally drew me back into myself. I remembered that when they were still together, we'd wheeled a shopping cart piled with toys out of the store and stuffed them all into the trunk and drove away without paying. *That was a fun day,* I was thinking, as I wrapped my arms around her legs while the cops took notes.

Chapter 4

The River

The summer I was five, we drove north, almost all the way to Canada, to see my mother's family, who gathered every summer on the St. Lawrence River.

When we arrived, we turned down a long driveway through scrubby woods until it ended at a huge lawn bordered by a curvy stone wall; beyond the wall was a wide river. We stopped in front of a big brown shingled house with sloping yellow awnings like eyelashes. I kicked off my shoes and silently greeted the life-size twin reindeer lawn sculptures, bypassed the house, and gained speed as I ran down the narrow stone path, skimming my hand along the rough lichen on all the pink rocks that bordered the paths and pushed up through the ground all around the island and from under the river.

I knew I had been here before because I had seen it on video: my father, topless Brigid Berlin, my mother, my youngest aunt, Chrissy, and me as a bald baby—all of us on the dock. The Thousand Islands, they called it. Or the River.

But I didn't have any real memories of my time there, only video ones.

I slowed myself down as I approached the dock and stopped next to the big boathouse on the bay. From there I searched the length of the dock for my aunts, excited to be smothered with attention by all five of my mother's sisters: Jeannie, Marybeth, Barb, Maureen, and Chrissy.

Some had their long limbs draped over the you'll-crack-your-head-on-the-edge diving board, some were dozing off, bare chested, wearing crocheted bikini bottoms, and trying to catch the fleeting spots of sun in between the shady spots from a swaying cypress tree.

My approaching footsteps revived them, and they all came rushing toward me—long, thin, and bony—spindly arms reaching out, cooing over my beauty, stroking my skin, hair tickling my face. Their breath smelled like breast milk.

I picked out Jeannie's lanky frame from the group and slithered into her arms. I had been weaned recently, but I still missed it so I sucked my thumb and giggled and fell limp under her touch like a sleepy puppy. My mother was the firstborn, Jeannie second. She lived on a ranch in Argentina and was currently my favorite aunt. Because she couldn't have babies of her own, and I was one of the firstborn, she was obsessed with me.

My mother approached her sisters, and the rest of them rose and gathered around her, laughing and screaming "Sue!" this and "Sue!" that.

I wondered who Sue was.

Nestling my face in Jeannie's hot, sun-tanned chest, I listened to all the sisters talking to one another with their peculiar drawl, just like my mother's. As they talked, they tickled my back and toyed with my hair. *I had gotten sooo big*, they said, *sooo sweet, sooo chahming. Look at my sweeeet little bottom.*

Chrissy, who was barely in her twenties, a Goldie Hawn look-alike, smiled and winked at me.

Marybeth, closer to my mother's age, was the exotic gap-toothed beauty; she stood on the diving board with her low-slung bikini bottom barely held up by her hip bones, and said, "Come on, Sue, let's get the little chickie in the boat before the sun goes down!"

"Who is Sue?" I finally asked. It was my mother's real name, apparently: Janet Susan Mary Hoffmann.

Once I was in the boat with the wind on my face and my orange life preserver and the up-down rhythm of the bow, I became hypnotized.

Chrissy gritted her teeth together and pushed the throttle all the way down. "We'll zoom right under the bridge!" she called out over the rev of the motor.

About a mile down current from the dock, the Thousand Islands Bridge spanned the distance from us to the mainland; cars looked like little bugs steadily crossing back and forth. Underneath the bridge, the steel blue Seaway was shadowed black and still, but then suddenly glittering and rippling as it unfurled toward us, expanding in width until we passed through its shadow—there it was, eighty feet above our heads—and then we were spit back into the sun, zooming on the glittering water again, past island after island, until eventually we were below the long stone wall at the end of the lawn, where the land looked like a rock cake with a slice cut out.

I looked up. Grandpa had built the wall so we kids wouldn't fall off the edge of lawn and into the deep river here, he said, and be swept up by the current and pulled to our deaths, or chopped to bloody bits by the ferocious boat propellers, or severed in half by the rusty steel hull of ships, the captain unaware that he had just mutilated a child's body. Slimy river moss grew from the rocks like long strands of emerald-green hair swirling in the current.

Chrissy let the boat drift past the big brown and white trimmed wraparound porch, and just past the house the circle of flags appeared—the American flag at its center—flapping and clinking. In front of the flags was the life-size statue of the Virgin Mary.

I loved this statue. I caught a glimpse of Mary's head as we passed her—her eyes seemed to follow me down the channel. Once Chrissy docked the boat, I extricated myself from the hands, ropes, and cleats and ran up the back hill to find her.

I stared at her stone face with the little curves at the corners of her mouth where her cheeks puffed out and appeared soft. The *Virgin* Mary. Somehow this was related to a *Bloody* Mary, I suspected. Or a Shirley Temple, which was a *Virgin* drink. She was taller than I was, and her concrete was old and cracked. A thin brown film covered her eyes, and between her fingers, spiders were at work building webs that draped alongside her gown and stretched outward past her toes and into the geraniums. Mary's hill was abandoned by the rest of the family—only Grandpa fiddled with the flagpoles and tended to the flowers around her feet where the light switches were hidden. I reached out and touched her hand before I ran into the house.

"Not so fast now . . . crack a head open," Grandpa said to me when I stumbled in.

His lips began quietly moving as he resumed counting the china in the big glass cabinet at the head of the dining room table. "Where the hell is the third set of the blue teacups, darn it all?" He turned around and peered down at me. "Did they fuss with my cabinets? I'm telling those girls for the last time."

But then he chuckled, picking me up. "Don't start hunching your back now, gotta keep it straight. Hell! Ha! You look just like Great Uncle Soot, just like him . . . poor soul." He chuckled more as he chewed on his lower lip and set me back down. And then he started counting again.

"Oh, stop it, Bill." Grandma came over now and pulled me toward her. I hugged her and buried my face in the soft yellow sweater she wore. Her blond hair was cut short, and the fuzzy soft curls were held in place with a sweet-smelling hair spray.

"She looks nothing like that dead brother of yours," she said to him and winked at me with her watery blue eyes. "Don't listen to a word, Alexandra."

She brought me out to the hot slate patio where she liked to work on her crossword puzzle. It felt good there: the warm stones on my bare feet, the *clink clank* of the flags on the flagpoles behind Mary. I lay on my belly, cheek against the hot slate, and stuck my thumb in my mouth to watch the lines of fat ants crawl past.

"You are too old for that," Grandma said. "I have an idea."

She walked me back into the living room and put a glass bowl on the mantel above the big fireplace. She said for every day I didn't suck my thumb I'd get a quarter dropped into the bowl. My mother had already tried to coat my thumb with bitter-tasting stuff, and I had managed to suck it all off, but I told Grandma I'd give it a try anyway.

"Good girl," she said.

MY MOTHER WENT away for the night, and I took a hot bath with a couple of cousins, warming up after the cold river had chilled us all to the bone. Afterward, wrapped in towels, we kids lounged around the upstairs hall on the green carpeting and the house lights went on and the kitchen started steaming and smelling good. All my aunts disappeared into their rooms to change.

I slid down the carpeted stairs, giving myself a rug burn, looking at the brown horse-and-carriage wallpaper. On this lower landing there was a window that opened up into the den, where we watched TV.

I watched the men through the glass.

Uncle Johnny was in there with Grandpa staring at the green golf fields flickering, listening to the smooth monotone of the announcer, and clinking the ice cubes in their cocktails. Johnny was a doctor. He was very tall and skinny with a pockmarked face. Sometimes he was affectionate and funny—he would take my arm and sniff the inside of it up and down like a dog—but he also walked around the house looking for warty cousins and forcing them to sit down while he burned off their warts with an electric contraption that made nasty, fleshy-smelling smoke.

Sitting on the stairs in front of the mirror, I let my thumb slip into my mouth, worried someone might catch me, like my cousin Franny, who might tattle on me when Grandma later asked me how my day went.

After a while, I went back upstairs, moving between the aunts' rooms. Suitcases were opened, clothes spilling out, makeup bags on the bureaus, open jars of Estee Lauder night cream, bottles of Guerlain and other eau de toilettes. Tinted pill bottles with pink and yellow capsules to help with sleep and burning pee. I draped myself over a bed and listened as my aunts laughed and whispered, moving around the lamp-lit room gracefully, mesmerizing me. I watched their faces in the bureau mirror as they drew the outlines of their own lips with a maroon pencil, wrapped silk scarves around their long necks, and sprayed perfume on their inner forearms. They talked about Aspen, Paris, and Argentina.

When I was close enough to Marybeth, I slipped a hand down her shirt and searched longingly for the source of that feathery-light pastry taste of breast milk. Marybeth let me have a nip. She was nursing her first baby, Oliver.

Soon my aunts scooped me up and we all went down to the dining room.

"How elegant," Barb, the ordinary-looking sister, said as she dimmed the lights and lit the candles.

"It's too damn dark in here," Grandpa complained. The candles made him grumpy.

During dinner, I slipped under the table, crawled past my aunts' painted toenails sticking out of their sandals like little candies, and tied Grandpa's feet together with his shoelaces.

Later, when he stood up and stumbled, I got so excited that I climbed on top of the table, clenched my fists, and clamped my jaw down so hard that my head trembled from the force.

"Oh, what a riot!" an aunt clapped her hands. My cheeks were trembling, and my toes were digging into the inside of my black patent leather Mary Janes.

"It's like she's going through heroin withdrawal!" Maureen, one of the youngest sisters, said. "Do it again, Allie!" she said, laughing.

So I did.

THAT NIGHT, I missed my mother so much it made my legs ache. I would have done anything to wrap them around her hips and nestle my face in her bony chest. I tiptoed into Grandma and Grandpa's room. She and Grandpa slept in separate beds on opposite sides of the room, each with a floral bedspread and a pink headboard. Above each headboard a colorful bleeding Christ was nailed to a wooden crucifix. A white wicker nightstand held a stack of *Reader's Digests*, a bible, a ceramic frog holding a parasol, and a set of rosary beads.

Grandma had to lift me into her bed because it was too high for me to climb up onto. She took one of my legs into her warm, wrinkled hands and rubbed it. I sucked my thumb and she didn't notice. From her bed I could hear Grandpa snoring and see past his lumpy body and out the window to where the gray reindeer were still standing on the front lawn in a pool of murky yellow light.

My mother said that when she was a teenager, he used that window to spy on her. I wished for her to appear on the lawn.

THE NEXT DAY my mother returned. The sisters merged together like birds flying in formation, coming apart, then together again, surrounding me, sending me into another blissed-out state.

But when they parted, I stayed close to my mother. Her pitch and tone were different from the others'. She seemed to know some kind of secret information that set us apart from them, and even though I was concerned about missing something over there with them, I couldn't leave her.

I thought it would make my mother laugh if I asked Grandma if I could "rub my tummy" as my mother's guru Muktananda suggested. When Grandma said, "Of course, honey, go right ahead," I straddled the back of the couch and started humping it. Grandma turned red and shaky.

"Go do that in your room," she snapped.

I hadn't expected it would upset her as much as it did. I examined my mother's face: Was she laughing? Not exactly. I crawled up the stairs and lay on my belly on the middle landing, looking through the slats in the railing. Down below, my aunts sat at the big round coffee table with a map of the River and all the islands painted on top. They looked like they were using the map to navigate a mysterious journey.

But then a sister left the navigation party and stormed up the stairs, past me, and slammed a bedroom door. I ran down the stairs and climbed on my mother's lap, but she felt stiff and cold. She was yelling at Uncle Johnny.

I was separated from her and taken out to the porch on the shoulders of my distant adult cousin, Ann. Something terrible was definitely happening inside the house on the other side of the sheer curtains. Ann was clamping my legs over her shoulders with cold hands, pacing the veranda, back and forth, back and forth, singing in a distracted voice: "She'll be coming round the mountain when she comes, she'll be riding six white horses when she comes . . ." While she sang, I could only catch glimpses of the other bodies through the sheer curtains. They all moved into the poolroom, which I could see through the windows at the other end of the porch, and suddenly Uncle Johnny was pushing my mother, then hovering over her.

I started to wriggle and squirm from Ann's shoulders, purposefully straining her neck. I dipped sideways, using all my body weight to force Ann to drop me. I ran into the house toward my mother. It felt like miles to get to her, running through sludge. Uncle Johnny's face was inches from hers.

As I ran toward her, I saw him pull back as if to hit her and I leaped, flying, it seemed, into her arms, and my head collided with his fist, making a strange dull thud.

Everyone surrounded us. Were they trying to help us or attack us? They were like a coven of possessed gargoyles. We untangled ourselves and escaped through the front door, ran down to the dock, and my mother used the boathouse phone to call a friend before we slunk to the floor, trembling, our breathing heavy.

Beyond the boathouse the River was empty and black except for the lights of the bridge that glinted green on the slivers of moonlight. Our breath wisped through the hollow inside returning back to us like invisible sprites.

A small motorboat soon disturbed the quiet of the bay and pulled up to the dock. A friend had arrived to take us away to their tiny island. My mother and I huddled together in the back of his boat, wind whipping up our hair, comforting each other, exhausted after the clash.

As the boat skidded along the black glass, I imagined all of them sitting up there in the glow of the living room, long legs crossed, shins kicking out rhythmically, shaking their heads about us and our crazy ways before they calmly returned to what my mother called their "ridiculous bourgeois behavior."

Fuck them, I thought.

Now

It's early in the morning and my mother walks into our bedroom. I'm pretending to still be asleep, but I crack an eye open to watch her. She looks out the window.

The old stone houses in Mount Airy are big. They have porches and fireplaces. Friends from New York think we live in the suburbs. This is technically the city, I tell them. The house across the lawn is almost the same as ours, but with a slightly different layout, and when we first moved here from the West Village, we watched the retired couple go about their daily business. Their kids went to the same Quaker school our kids are now going to. A few weeks later, in the middle of the night, we stood at our bedroom window, red ambulance lights dancing on our faces, and watched as they slipped the dead husband into the hatch. Our future, I thought.

I was nervous about my mother seeing this house. I knew she would think there was enough room for her to move in.

She turns her attention from the window to our bed, walking closer to examine the scene.

Miko still sleeps in between Nick and me, naked, skin against skin, his foot perfectly fit into the curve of my waist and hip; an arm draped over Nick's chest; an extension of us; or us, an extension of him.

I feel little prickles of shame over this display of intimacy she is still examining. At least it's Miko I'm wrapped up with and not Nick. If Nick had his arm draped over me, I would push it off as soon as I heard the floor creak under her footsteps.

The very first time she met Nick, twenty-five years ago, we were in bed together. I was hiding behind his back—hiding from her—in his apartment in Tivoli, off campus. I had just graduated from Bard College and he had another year or so left. She and I had argued the night before, and she stormed out of my apartment and onto the streets of Tivoli, where she paced and ranted for what seemed like hours.

While she was ranting, I snuck out and used the shadows to escape, unseen, into Nick's place, directly behind mine.

By morning she had found us. As students, we never locked our doors in this little town on the Hudson, so I heard her marching in, calling my name, my heart racing as her footsteps ascended the stairs, and then there she was, barging into his bedroom, still furious, still ranting.

Nick said: "Get out. You're a dictator just like my father."

I was silent and stunned, slinking lower behind his back.

You never yell back at Viva, I thought, right then eternally devoting myself to him.

I open my eyes now.

I don't want to hear her talk about how I have what she doesn't—this king-size bed, these linen sheets, this husband. The husband really irks her.

We joke, joke that she would be thrilled if Nick died. She would slip right into this big bed with Miko and me and try to coax from me all the ills of my long marriage.

She fingers the sheets.

"Wow, these are really nice, honey, where'd you get them?"

Anything you say—and I mean anything—can and will be used against you. Eventually. Even if twenty years pass with no mention of the tidbit of information you gave up, you can't relax. She'll always be holding the tidbit close, ready to use it when the time is right.

If I were to say something negative about Nick, it would be like blood for a vampire. But even something offhand about the expensive linen sheets could be used to snare me.

I know exactly where I got this bedding, but I say, "I'm not sure. I can't remember."

She looks at us and laughs.

I think, for a moment, she is appreciating the cuteness, but no, there is something sinister in the laugh.

"You've really got the Messiah complex with Miko," she says.

Ah, so that's what she's getting at.

"Yup, guess so," I say to my mother in my usual way, void of emotion.

To deny or to defend is to admit vulnerability. "We better get ready to go to the meeting," I say.

"It's called *Meeting for Worship*," Nick corrects. "It's not AA."

My mother shoots me a raised eyebrow—she wants me to ridicule Nick with her, to bond over what she thinks is his arrogance, his desire to correct.

I look away.

Chapter 5

Argentina

When I was six, my mother and I visited Aunt Jeannie in Argentina, at her husband Cuco's ranch in Córdoba.

Soon after we arrived, my mother took off, and I stayed behind.

I eased into Jeannie's arms as though the terrible thing at the River had never happened.

Every night I stayed with her, she would anoint me, like a living saint. She'd sit by the bath and gently scrub me all the way down to the soles of my feet until I was tingly and pink. She combed my hair until it was fluffy and then sprinkled perfumed powder on my damp skin. When she got excited about her love for me, she would grind her teeth together and move her lower jaw slightly askew from her upper jaw while she spoke to me in a baby voice. She made little whiny spasmodic noises while she hugged and kissed me.

Every morning I'd join Jeannie and Cuco in their bedroom at one end of the long ranch house, their legs outlined and tucked tightly under the crisp bedsheets and pinned under two bamboo breakfast trays that were delivered by the housekeeper. I was invited to wedge in between them and share their food—soft-boiled eggs with evenly cut toast strips, slices of fried jambon, dulce de membrillo, pastries, and coffee with frothy milk.

After the housekeeper took the trays away, I'd hold my breath while Jeannie flipped her skinny long legs over the side of the bed and winced in pain as her feet touched the floor and she slowly allowed her body weight to descend.

Two years before, while she was sweeping dead leaves by the empty pool, she fell into it, landing standing up on the concrete in the empty deep end, shattering both her heels. Because of this, maybe, she seemed older than my mother.

Even though I was only six, I could tell Jeannie had a delicate air about her, a brittleness, like if you hugged her too hard, you'd crack her.

ONE NIGHT, my mother called and said, "Honey, say hello to *Bob*."

The reception was scratchy, but I could still hear that particularly enlivened tone she got when she was happy about a man. I could imagine the warm flush on her skin.

Bob?! I thought, *Who the hell is he?* The name *Bob* infuriated me. *No, I don't want to say hello to Bob.*

He got on the phone. He sounded like a robot: "Hello, Alexandra."

No one called me *Alexandra*. Pretending to be nice to him was like having my nails pulled off.

When she got back on the phone, I tried to inject some life into my voice. "Where are you now?" I asked her.

"Honey, I'm flying. We're flying over Arches National Park. In Bob's plane. It's fabulous. I'll be there soon."

So that's where she has been, I thought. *Flying in some plane with a fool.* I imagined her in a mini silver plane, her hair blowing, zooming underneath arches, like a scene in a Bugs Bunny cartoon.

When my mother came back—no Bob to be seen, thank God— we rode a black stallion together. The horse galloped so fast that we were afraid we might slip off his heaving back, slick with sweat, but his feet drove into the earth until he suddenly seemed to float and we floated too, just above his arching spine, laughing and whooping.

Later that day, during dinner, my mother argued with the rest of Cuco's family about guerrilla warfare and fascists. While they were yelling, I accidentally sliced my heel open on the edge of a swinging door, and there was a flap of skin hanging off. Jeannie rushed for iodine and whisked me into the same bathroom she had been anointing me in every evening before my mother had arrived.

"All this political jabber. We don't need it, you and me," Jeannie whispered to me as she bandaged my heel.

I prayed Jeannie would not malign my mother. We could still hear her in the dining room: "They're torturing innocent people right across the street!" she yelled.

"You don't know that," someone yelled back.

"I know something is going on when there are men with machine guns guarding a warehouse—guns everywhere! How can you deny it? It's guerrilla warfare!"

I wanted to tell Jeannie that I agreed with my mother and that I loved Che Guevara too, but instead I let her rub calendula oil on my feet.

That night my mother was wound up, pacing the room. "The Ferreyras are pretending they don't know what's going on. That's the worst crime of all! I mean they brag about how Che came to the ranch to visit Chichina . . . did you know that? . . . And then they act like fascists."

I nodded my head yes, but even though I loved Che, I didn't really know anything about him or Chichina. Sometimes my mother thought that I knew more than I did; I preferred it that way. I figured I would eventually find out who these characters were.

She continued, "Well, Che came here to visit Cuco's aunt—they were in love—so they brag about that, you know; because they are related to Chichina, they feel they're related to Che. Che! One of the greatest revolutionaries of our time! And then they deny the fascism right under their noses!"

Finally, my mother calmed down and we fell asleep together.

The next morning there was a loud pounding on our bedroom door. I had been dreaming that the pounding sound was gorillas (not guerrillas) coming to torture us.

When I woke, my mother was already sitting up, hypnotized, staring at the chandelier that was swinging back and forth above her head. Cuco's face was in the window. He was frantically motioning for us to come outside. Out there in the misty air the entire pool shifted in the earth until its concrete foundations cracked. The crack echoed down the ranch, and the ground swayed under my feet. The maids ran outside yelling, *Dios mío! Dios mío!* The horses whinnied in the distance, huffing through their nostrils, and pounding their hooves.

An earthquake.

It was time to leave.

Chapter 6

On the Road Again

When we arrived at JFK from Argentina, we ended up sharing a cab with a man who brought us to his apartment to spend the night. I saw a pretty bowl of oranges arranged in a perfect triangular pile sitting on a black-varnished countertop. Something was wrong about how neat his place was. My mother said that overly neat people were disturbed.

He juggled those oranges, two, three, even five perfect orange globes hovering in midair passing one another at the top of an invisible arc. He said it was a trick of the eye and tried to teach me how to do it—something about an orange having to always pass from one hand to the other. I was appreciative of the fact that he was trying to engage me, but I could never manage the oranges. (Even so, I would later try to show off and teach people to juggle oranges based on this one faulty lesson.)

That evening, my mother tucked me into the big bed in the only bedroom, and I quickly realized that they had made a bed for themselves in the living room. She was up to no good again. *I will not let her sleep with that man*, I thought to myself.

I begged her to fall asleep with me, clung to her, wrapped my legs around her hips, my arms around her body. The moment she thought I had dozed off, she snuck back into the other room. *How was it possible that this circus fool could be drawing her attention away from the warmth of my body?* It was unthinkable. *Unbearable.*

I tried to be patient, tried to wait it out, but the torment was too much. I lasted only thirty seconds at most. I slipped out of bed, tiptoed behind her, and was assaulted with the sight of their large makeshift bed strewn on the floor of his living room, flickering in the candlelight.

"What are you doing?" I asked, standing still, like a possessed kid ghost. She cajoled me back into the bedroom, slipped me into the bed, tried to appease me. I heard and felt how enlivened she was, how easygoing. The warm flush on her skin destroyed me.

She was relentless.

But so was I.

I kept the vigil all night. Every time she left me, I'd walk straight into their living room and insist that she escort me back to bed while I envisioned suffocating the man with his oranges and setting his hair on fire with the candle flame.

Soon after that night we began to roam again.

ASPEN.

We were driving over mountains, the car stuttering almost to a stop as we crested the peaks, and then gaining speed as we descended.

"I never should have given Bob's number to Marybeth—all that could have been ours. Oh, *how* could I have? I should have known! All my sisters have *always* stolen my boyfriends—that's why I first moved to New York. To get away from them. And then they followed me here! *All that could have been ours . . .*"

"All what?"

Here we go again . . .

"The planes, this house in Aspen . . ." she said.

"*Bob*," he said when we arrived, formally introducing himself, nodding with a huge toothy smile and vigorously shaking my hand, "Bob Fulton, thank you, thank you."

This man who was greeting me at the door was *Bob*—the very same man my mother was fixated on when I was in Argentina, the same man who flew my mother under the arches. He was now, apparently, my aunt Marybeth's boyfriend, and Marybeth was pregnant with his kid. Marybeth didn't seem to mind that my mother and Bob were once together and that now they seemed to be the best of friends.

Why had the Fates cursed me to contend with this interloper?

Bob had a shock of grayish-blond hair that swooped over his forehead and covered one eye. He wore rose-tinted glasses with large square frames *inside* (apparently he was sensitive to light); he must have been at least seven feet tall with broad bony shoulders and a square chin.

Jesus Christ, I thought, *he's worse than he sounded on the phone.*

He carried around a tiny book about being in "the Now."

Fuck the Now, I thought.

IN BED THAT NIGHT, my mother whispered to me: "See, honey? All this could have been ours. I should have married Bob. But I couldn't keep kissing those cold lips. Damn it, I just knew I shouldn't have given him MB's number. We could have had this beautiful house."

I thought about the way Bob played the saxophone, which, to my horror, the women seemed to love, and how he left poems around the house written with a black felt-tip pen on white unlined paper, capital letters all the exact same size, evenly spaced. I thought about how he always sported a huge smile that exposed his upper row of teeth, made deep creases in his cheeks, and crinkled his eyes in the corners. No matter how many times I saw him, he would greet me with that smile and extend a stiff right arm, shake my hand, squint his eyes behind the rose-tinted glasses, nod his head rhythmically up and down, and repeat my name over and over again: "Alex, Alex, Alex, yes, yes . . . thank you . . . yes. Good to see you."

I also thought about how he would always say, "Yes, thank you," even though I did nothing for him to be thankful for and, in fact, I wanted to ruin his life for first taking my mother's attention and then my aunt's.

Why can't these women see he's a psychopath?!

"I hate Bob. He's yucky," I said.

"You're right. He *is* yucky. But maybe I should have just tried to bear through it, so we could have had this great house."

"No! He's disgusting. I can't even stand to look at him. I told you—we should move back to the Chelsea."

"Shh!," she said, worried they might hear me. "Well, good then. I'm glad I didn't marry him . . ."

And then there was a long pause, and I could feel her thoughts rumbling, percolating to the top until she was compelled to say more, however weak the delivery was.

"But maybe you could have learned to love him—"

"No!" I *had* to act very decisively or else she wouldn't stop regretting.

"We could have lived in—"

"No!" I slammed my fist down on the pillow.

"I really should have—"

"Never! No more coulda, shoulda, woulda!"

BOLINAS.

We left Bob's house and continued driving.

In order to redirect her attention from lamenting about Bob, I improvised a country song and sang it in a southern accent: "Oh, men are such fools, and the women don't see how they look like such ghouls; oh, women you take so much time, and oh, you sure do seem so dumb not to see how they really are truly such scum . . ."

We continued along the winding blacktop until it just barely licked the edge of dramatic ocean cliffs and ended at a little house perched above roiling waves.

An old friend of my mother's and her daughter, Chandra, had moved to this small town above San Francisco and helped us find this shack on a cliff where my mother could work on a screenplay about Elvis's sad life.

She hated driving around Bolinas, and every time we went somewhere, she'd stop periodically to catch her breath. "Oh, God, honey, don't look down there. I have such vertigo. Ooo! Those idiots just speeding by! I have a child in the car, for God's sake."

This fearfulness annoyed me.

Her continued fixation on Bob also annoyed me.

The ocean pummeled the rocks below our fragile shack.

I had been excited to hang out with Chandra, but she and her friends quickly decided I was weird—maybe because of the blue granny glasses I had to wear after the eye operation (I thought they were cool), or because I made up songs (my mother thought they were genius), or because I sometimes humped things in public (I thought this was funny).

I began to secretly bide my time until my aunt Chrissy's green convertible arrived. She lived in San Francisco and would often invite me to her apartment for weekend visits. We would leave the Bolinas house full of giddy enthusiasm, silk scarves tied around our heads, confidently speeding along the cliff edges listening to Rod Stewart.

Chrissy lived with her older husband, John, in a fancy apartment. She was barely twenty-five and already pregnant with her first child. We would relax, naked, on her zebra skin rug in front of the fireplace and sing "If You Think I'm Sexy" in husky voices. I admired her pregnant belly while she rubbed the tight skin with cocoa butter to ward off stretch marks. Her whole life felt so much cleaner and brighter than the one I had with my mother—with our mattress on the floor surrounded by ramshackle walls.

One weekend when I returned home, my mother was irritable. "It was your idea to come here and now all you want to do is get away."

"I don't want to get away," I mumbled. She seemed so mean suddenly. I just wanted to have fun with Chrissy. *Did I want to get away from her?* I wondered.

"You begged me to move here to be close to Chandra," my mother said.

That's true, I thought. *But now Chandra hates me.* I didn't want to tell her because she might get mad at Chandra's mother.

"I got us this beautiful house so you'd be near Chandra, and instead you go to Chrissy's every weekend."

I vowed to stay close and prove I did love Bolinas, prove I didn't want to get away.

But when Chrissy suggested taking me to the River while my mother continued working, my resolve disintegrated. I tried to hide my excitement because my mother had said she was never going back after what happened with Uncle Johnny. I knew I should vow to never return as well, but being with all the aunts and cousins seemed like heaven.

I told my mother I didn't want to leave her.

Then she said, "No, go ahead; go and see your cousins. Maybe I'll meet you there. I could paint," and I realized she had begun to let go of the grudge as well.

I packed desperately, trying not to appear too eager to get away. I knew she would be alone above the ocean, writing about how Elvis shit in his bed because he drank too much and took too many pills and how his maid had to clean it all up for him. I tried not to look at her.

While I was packing, she said, "I always let you do exactly what you want."

Did she? I wondered. I was too worried she was thinking about changing her mind to examine this any further.

"I know," I said. "You're the best mom."

Frantic, but pretending to be reluctant, I dragged my blue suitcase into the living room. It was as big as I was. It just sat there, like a dumb thug.

"I'll really miss you," I said, searching for the green MG to appear in the driveway.

Chapter 7

Tribeca

I had a wonderfully uneventful time at the River without my mother. As the summer ended, I was back on the road with her until we eventually found ourselves lying on my father's bed in his new loft in Tribeca. I was happy to be back in New York, though we had nowhere to live.

The sun was setting, darkening the loft. Michel was sitting in a chair by his desk at the foot of the bed, fiddling with something on his video camera and telling my mother how he was going to build a wall with Bob, his roommate, to make me my own room.

I loved this huge L-shaped loft. Bob's half was in the back, over an old firehouse on Varick Street, and Michel's side faced White Street. It was bright and neat. Michel had a bed and a couch by the windows, and on the other side of the room was his studio—a few small tube TV monitors, various editing equipment with silver knobs and spools of tape, and shelves neatly stacked with black plastic VHS cases with white labels: Morocco, Viva on the Phone, The Chelsea 1973, Zuma Beach.

I was going to stay there while my mother looked for our next place to live.

"Fine," she said after he delivered the news about my own room. She flared her nostrils and looked out the window. "But I hope you're not using anymore."

He looked into the camera lens.

My mother said she just wanted me to be happy.

"I already am happy," I replied.

"So good. She stays wiz me, zen," my father said.

"We don't have any money," my mother said with a sigh.

"I pay."

"Come on." She laughed. "You don't have a cent! Why don't you just get a job driving a cab?"

I squirmed, praying she would leave before a fight started.

"Oh, Viva," he said, exasperated. "We figure it out, OK?"

"Easy for you to say who has never had a job his entire life."

"I hate Reagan," I interjected.

We had just been to a communist lesbian meeting, and I knew this would make her laugh. It worked. "I do too, honey, he's a pig," she said, relenting slightly.

After she left, I watched her from the window, walking across West Broadway. A garbage can blew over the curb and rolled to the gutter. She turned her head up to the window and waved at me. She must have sensed me watching.

That moment reminded me of *An Unmarried Woman,* a movie starring Jill Clayburgh, which we were both obsessed with. Jill's character vomits after learning that her husband is having an affair. She has to start a new life, single in Soho, meeting men, and discovering her independence. My mother and I had hooted and hollered over the vomit scene, ridiculing how melodramatic it was. And yet the movie moved me. It captured the empty garbage-y streets of downtown and the way women cried at their little kitchen tables about the men who abandoned them, how they collapsed, were laid up in bed, said they couldn't do it all.

I blew her a kiss back, and she continued to Church Street to search for a cab. I felt terrible watching her leave but soon turned my attention to the loft.

My father reminded me to be careful around the editing table, where there was videotape threaded between various spools, moving so fast it looked still.

"Don't ever touch the exposed tape," he said.

When he left the room, I pointed my index finger as close to the exposed tape as I could, wanting to feel it move, to test it.

"Arrêt!" he snapped when he returned, catching me. Startled, I pulled my finger back and tried not to cry. His moods were unfamiliar after the long journey without him. He must have sensed that I was shaken and tried to soothe me by playing videos from when we lived together in the Chelsea. I settled in front of the monitor and began to draw while I watched myself being born, nursing, toddling through the lobby, being held by the big-boobed white-haired operator in front of the old-fashioned operator's booth.

The good old days, I thought.

Later he tucked me into his bed and massaged my feet.

"Don't suck!" he chastised.

I wiped my wet thumb on his sheets.

Later still, he got into bed with me and before he pulled up the edge of the top sheet and secured it between his teeth, he said, "Bon nuit, mon cheri, fete de bon rêve, à demain." And that's how he slept: naked except for a silk scarf and the sheet between his teeth.

I SOON DISCOVERED that Michel also had an aura of loneliness, but unlike Viva, his was unspoken; he hunched over his studio desk and crinkled and clicked his paraphernalia.

What exactly he was doing was a mystery at the time—one that I could only loosely piece together with the evidence I had seen throughout the years: drawers in his desk with rolled-up dollar bills, burned pieces of tinfoil, razor blades. Little things burned to brown.

While he did it, I would become deliberately absorbed in a line on the page of a book, or the flickering black-and-white images of the television show *The Electric Company*, or pulling my hair tightly back into a yellow plastic barrette. These moments of self-imposed insulation and concentration—a willfulness to *not*-know what was plainly in front of me—did not normally last very long though. Minutes, maybe.

So I prolonged each minute as much as I could, making the passing of this time appear natural, like I would always take this exact amount of time to do my hair.

I wanted him to think I was oblivious.

After the crinkling stopped, he stepped across the threshold, I stepped across the threshold, and we reentered reality together. He would rub his pinkie finger under his upper lip, begin working or making dinner, and we would both continue like those minutes had never existed.

I let him have this secret.

MY MOTHER FINALLY FOUND us an apartment in NYC, but it didn't last long. It was a small loft-like space that her friend Steve Mass, who owned the Mudd Club, was renting us. Our windows looked over the 8th Street Playhouse, where the characters from *The Rocky Horror Picture Show* loitered, waiting for one of the shows to start.

"This is so much better than that dump of a hotel," she said.

I pretended to agree, but the apartment didn't feel right to me.

For some months I alternated between the Eighth Street loft, my father's loft, and my friend Zoe's loft.

I had met Zoe at my new school in the West Village, PS 3, where I quickly fell in love with her. She was beautiful—long silky black hair, hooded eyelids, a little bow-shaped mouth—and she had a mischievous side, like me.

Zoe's mother, Judy, loved and looked just like Bettie Page, and painted portraits of Castro. She and Viva got along great. They would sit around the lofts for hours talking about what fucking assholes men were (including Zoe's father).

While the women talked and laughed, Zoe and I played our "party" games: We were "wild girls," desperate for a sniff or a smoke. We stuffed socks into our flimsy DIY "bras," rolled up a dollar bill and pretended to sniff salt or air—cutting it with a razor, smoking it, sticking a pinkie finger in a nostril and rubbing it underneath an upper lip, against the gums. "Oh, yeah, man . . . ," we would say, leaning back in ecstasy. "That's gooooood. Good stuff."

Free women, enjoying a wild night out.

Once Judy called my mother, crying, after a fight with Zoe's father, and we brought her to the ER with a deep puncture wound in her arm. I didn't mind the ER. We recently had to take an old friend of my mother's to Bellevue for talking to imaginary people in the gutter, and I enjoyed watching all the crazy ladies in the waiting room.

That night, while they stitched up Judy's arm, Zoe and I played Mr. Bill, a game inspired by a *Saturday Night Live* bit, which revolved around making miniature worlds out of clay—in the ER room it was pieces of pretzels the nurse gave us—and violently crushing them.

Meanwhile, my mother tried to make Judy feel better about being married to a prick: "The only reason Michel wanted to get married was so he could film it, so the wedding scene could be part of the movie we were already making together. But we had a huge fight because he kept saying we couldn't have the ceremony until he found a floodlight and film . . . and he slapped me when I complained! Well, I did kick him first . . . and none of the film went through! None! He wouldn't even wear a ring . . ."

Judy laughed with my mother, and they both agreed that all men were pricks. Zoe and I loved our fathers despite their shortcomings, but we didn't mind our mothers' laughing at their expense.

THE YEAR WE WERE SEVEN, Zoe and I decided to be Green Olives for Halloween. My mother used a tangle of chicken wire and made a frame that fit over my entire body, bending it as she went along into a huge, hollow oval. I was impressed with how clever she was.

When I went to bed the night before Halloween, she was still wrapping long strips of sticky wet cheesecloth around the wire. Before I fell asleep I told her not to worry too much about it.

In the middle of the night she woke me up.

"I don't know, honey," she said. "I think the eyes are too low. You won't be able to see. Get in it and try."

"It'll be fine," I mumbled.

She insisted I get up and do a fitting, and decided that the eyes had to be changed. Nothing could redirect her attention.

"You better get some sleep," I reminded her, but she continued to work on it.

By the time I woke up for school, she had created a magnificent costume—a hollow, dark green shell with two holes for my eyes. It was big. So big that the sides scraped against the doorway. She stood back and examined it.

"It's a little wrinkled," she said, tilting her head as she inspected it, as though she were looking at a painting in a museum. "I think it looks more like a *Greek* olive."

I put it over my head and looked through the eyeholes.

"Let me add some black to it," she insisted.

While she painted it, I sang from the inside, my voice muffled, "I'm a *black Greek olive*—and I luv ya so," and I did a little soft-shoe dance.

That afternoon my father picked up Zoe and me from school to take us trick-or-treating through the West Village. He trailed us as we squeezed our olive costumes into restaurants and apartment buildings. By the end of the night the olives had taken a hammering. They were falling apart and I was ready to be freed. My father was frustrated by the cumbersome structure, and he finally snapped, "Dis fucking sing, dump it!"

But as I tossed the tangle of wire and paper into a garbage can in Washington Square Park, I had a bad feeling.

The next day when I returned from school, my mother was frantic.

"Where's the olive?"

I tried to quickly think up a lie, but nothing came to mind.

"Goddamn him!" she shrieked. "He is just so irresponsible! He has *always* done that! Just *dumped* things when he got sick of them. In Europe he would rent cars, total them, and then just *dump* them on the side of the road!"

I told her there was no way I could have brought it back to school, that I was the one who wanted to throw it out—not him—but she was already calling him to yell at him.

Now

My mother is pacing the playground on the Quaker school campus wearing an old Indiana Jones kind of hat and a full-length dark brown Australian Outback coat. We are waiting to go into the Meeting House.

Many layers live underneath this getup. Each one has a different sartorial vibe: pastel cashmeres, threadbare Dries van Noten harem pants, and Eileen Fisher—like linen drapey stuff with a base of silk long johns and Uggs. Paint splatters complete the look.

"That's stupid," Miko is telling another kid at the Quaker school playground.

"*Stupid* is a bad word; we don't say that word," the kid informs Miko.

"Well, that's *really* stupid," my mother chimes in. She loves to argue with little kids. I hide my laughter as she sits down on the bench next to me and whispers, "I just loathe it when parents tell their kids they can't say certain words—don't you? It's so fucking stupid."

"I know," I whisper back.

"What's worse," I add, "is that some of the families have a 'swear jar,' and if you say *fuck*, you have to put a dollar in the jar!"

"No! No, no!" she says, covering her eyes in horror.

"Yeah, there is nothing worse than a seven-year-old little goody-two-shoes fuckface telling you that you have to pay her to curse."

"Eww! Oh, how awful!! What about the parents who refuse to . . . what is it called . . . *gender* their kids?! Can you be*lieve* it?!"

I glance over my shoulder to see if anyone has heard. The problem with getting her going is that she starts to say offensive things. I try to shush her and suggest that, on the subject of gender, it is healthier to adjust to modern times.

"Oh my God, don't be ridiculous! I was the *queen* of the fags!"

Again, I glance over my shoulder, and then we gather up Miko and head toward the Meeting House.

When we left NYC because we couldn't afford it anymore, we moved the kids from PS 3 (my old public school) to this school, where Nick had gone, and absorbed its Quaker values. But that was a long time ago, and we weren't sure what it would be like now. When we arrived, Nick and I were both stunned by what seemed like a colder, more calculating, buttoned-up vibe than what we were used to in New York.

"If you are called to speak, Mom, go right ahead," I say as we walk together.

I'm excited to see how the room—full of well-intentioned people trying to practice simplicity, peace, integrity, community, equality, and stewardship—will hold Viva in the light. I love challenging a person's integrity with my mother.

As we enter the Meeting House, another parent is telling my mother how much their family adores their pets.

My mother looks at me and rolls her eyes.

"Well," she tells them, "I can't decide if the happiest day of my life was the day I lost interest in sex or the day my second dog died and I was finally free of dogs."

I look at the parent and make an exaggerated eek face.

Then my mother turns to me and says, "Don't worry, honey, I won't tell them you tried to kill me."

I pretend I didn't hear her and we sit in silence.

There is rustling and a cough here and there.

Miko and the other kids fidget.

It's true: in the past I have snapped. I have slid my hands through her hair and pulled, hard, my face inches from hers, locking in on her child-like blue eyes while I ferociously pin her down to the bed as I describe what I will do to her if she says another word, spitting the words into her ear: "I'll bash your fucking brains out."

What had she said to me in my house in Tivoli when I was a twentysome-thing woman? I can't even remember what made me try to kill her before another word escaped from her mouth and Nick had to pry me off her.

What did she say to me ten years later in the West Village house? Something that made me want to crack her skull open in front of little Lui just to make her stop saying the words.

If only I could tell the story in some cohesive way—in a she-said-this-then-that way—but when I try to grasp the actual sentences that she said, they slip through my fingers like beads of mercury.

I'm certain that if she and the Dalai Lama were locked in a cell to-gether, and she turned the screw on him, he would crack within the hour. He might even try to kill her because he has been kowtowed to his whole life and never forced to contend with a Viva. I've always suspected I'm more patient and loving than the great masters because I've been in a cell with her for a lifetime and have physically attacked her only twice.

It's true, I have reduced her to a cowering trot. Though while I was pinning her down, I did wonder if she was actually terrified or maybe just doing a rendition of Mina in *Nosferatu*—clutching her bosom, wide-eyed and stunned. When she wailed for the cops, I wondered if she knew she would end up with the upper hand. If she was holding on to the moment so she could say to me, much later, years and years later: "Don't worry, honey, I won't tell them you tried to kill me."

She stands up now, moved to speak.

Here we go, I think, bracing myself for her to throw me under the bus with a room full of Quakers.

"I was just meditating on how I'll be dead soon and how kids these days are not taught to respect their elders. In third world countries everyone lives together. Miko never listens to me. But men don't listen, so why should boys? One day he'll wake up and say, 'Shit, I wish I had been nicer to my grandmother.' But I'll be dead by then. Thank God."

Brilliant.

Chapter 8

Connecticut and Tribeca

Honey, wake up! We've got to protect the baby tomatoes!" My mother was frantic, jostling me awake. "There's a frost. Hurry!"

There was no escaping. I could hide under the toasty covers and pretend I didn't exist, but she wouldn't fall for that. I begrudgingly layered up and trudged behind her, into the frigid night, my frosty breath leading me forward like an angry ghost.

My mother had decided the city was unlivable after we had been robbed at the Eighth Street apartment. Her friend, the artist John Chamberlain, offered us his guesthouse in Essex, Connecticut. She was working on a new screenplay called *The Secret Life of Shakespeare* that Chamberlain had something to do with.

"Here, take these little bags and tie them around the plants, tight on the bottom. But not *too* tight. Oh, *God*, they're all going to die!" she was saying.

As I did as I was told I thought: *What the hell was I thinking wanting to move here? I hate gardens and two-story houses. I hate yards.*

It was clear I had made a terrible mistake.

When I found out the Essex house was big, had two bedrooms, a washer and dryer, a dishwasher, a small aboveground pool with a deck built around it so it looked like a real pool, and a large back-yard, I told my mother that I thought it was a great idea. We could get a dog! We would be like a sitcom family. Also, it was a short train ride to NYC.

But once we arrived, the land, the dog, and the house became burdens—entities that my mother had to contend with and I, some-how, was roped into the struggle to organize and dominate them. Just feeding the new dog was as stressful as if we were responsible for the lives of all earth's creatures. That dog was basically thirty pounds of guilt in a fur sack.

When we had arrived in Essex, my mother quickly set her sights on planting the perfect garden, but she soon discovered that the land was too sandy, so Chamberlain introduced her to Gary, a mush-room expert and a live-snake collector. I called him Country Gary to distinguish him from Gary Indiana, our very small, bug-eyed writer friend (whom I loved because he confided in me about the men he had sex with and often came to visit us in this new land so he and my mother could collaborate on *The Secret Life of Shake-speare*).

Country Gary helped her arrange for two truck beds full of black soil to be dumped into the backyard.

This night, my mother seemed completely unconcerned that my fingers would be lost to the frost. As I struggled to close the mouths of the little paper bags around the lower stems with strands of cook-ing twine, I fantasized about the coming weekend in Tribeca when I would be freed from the stress of my mother trying to tame the chaos of seasonal change. Or maybe, I was starting to suspect, my mother brought the chaos on herself.

In Tribeca I could do as I pleased: space out in the little bedroom my father had made for me; roam the streets; eat well-done filet mignon at the packed tables of One Fifth with my father and all his friends; and when the cigarette smoke stung my eyes too much, I could go out into the night air, hoist myself up into the nook where they kept the menu lit behind glass, and meditate on the empty, quiet breadth of lower Fifth Avenue.

When my mother was finally satisfied we had covered all the baby plants, she said we could go back to bed.

Once inside, I jammed myself back under the covers, fuming. I had never disagreed with her before, but I thought *this couldn't be right, waking up a child at two a.m. to save baby plants.*

From then on I tried my best to steer clear of the yard.

ON LATE AFTERNOONS in Essex, after ballet class, I would wander over to the main house, where John and his wife, Lorraine, lived, to get away from the gardening. I fit myself into the hollowed-out shapes of a block of foam that John had cut with a chain saw to make a sculptural couch. From the foam nooks, I watched *The Love Boat* and *Fantasy Island* until I began to worry that my mother might be getting agitated, whether due to my absence or just some asshole who had wronged us.

When I made my way back to the two-story house across the lawn, I'd settle myself in my room and listen to my three albums: *Grease, Silk Purse,* and *Parallel Lines.* As I examined their jackets (*Why is Linda sitting with the pigs?*), and obsessed over Debbie's hair and Sandy's bad-girl outfit, I kept an extra ear out for anything going awry downstairs.

One afternoon I was listening to the song "Will You Still Love Me Tomorrow" when she ran into the house calling up to me: "Don't go outside!"

I turned down the music and listened as she got on the phone with Country Gary. She told him that she noticed what she at first thought was a large brown umbrella, sitting open on the ground. As she approached, it began to move slowly away revealing a shallow pit filled with what looked like translucent Ping-Pong balls. Country Gary said our yard might be a breeding ground for snapping turtles. They're harmless, he said, unless you get in their way. If you do get in the turtle's way, he warned, and it snaps at you and takes hold . . . well, then it never lets you go—even if you decapitate it—its head will still be attached to whatever part of your body it had taken hold of.

My mother hung up and stood at the bottom of the stairs and called up to me: "Don't go outside! There's a giant snapping turtle—the biggest thing I've ever seen—it could take off your entire foot. Your leg, even! And even if we cut its head off, it would still be attached. Oh my God, honey, promise me: do *not* set foot outside."

Perfect, I thought. *Thank you, snapping turtle.*

For days afterward, my mother obsessed over the turtle. After she borrowed Country Gary's shotgun, she spent hours pacing back and forth in front of the garden, trying to decide whether she should shoot it.

"Shoo, shoo!" she'd yell with a shrill tone.

The turtle wouldn't budge.

One afternoon when I returned home she was stirring a pot of turtle egg soup. While the broth simmered, so did her guilt.

"Oh, Alex," she moaned. "It was probably harmless. Why did I let Country Gary give me that gun?"

I gave her a hug. "It's OK, Mom. I'm proud of you! You had to kill it, otherwise"—I had to remember why it was that she had to do it—*Oh, right*: "Otherwise, it could have taken off my leg and you'd have had to chop its head off and then pry my leg out of its mouth."

"You're right! Now you can play in the yard again."

I had to get up the nerve to ask the next question. "Actually . . . can you give me a ride to the station?" I tentatively asked her.

I had weekend plans in Tribeca, and I really couldn't afford her getting into a mood about this.

"Oh, that's why you're being so nice. So you can go see your perfect father. Sure, honey, I'll give you a ride."

Some minutes passed and I thought she had moved on. I started to head up to my bedroom to pack.

"Damn that Gary!" she shrieked as though Country Gary had just come in and poked her with a needle. "I never should have listened to him, goddamn it!"

At least, I thought, she was fixated on Country Gary and not my father.

I WAS GOING ON NINE, and life in Connecticut had become a tug of war between "the country"—where I was misunderstood, where my mother was beginning to more regularly drive me crazy, and where I couldn't wear my yellow stretchy pants and velour shirts because the kids gave me looks of disapproval—and "the city"—where there was a promise of adventure, and where my father would wait for me at Grand Central with his new French girlfriend, a wonderful young ballet dancer named Florence.

Florence was the opposite of the Unmarried Woman. She was joyous and freckled with plump lips that erupted into a cute gummy smile. She had big boobs—too big for professional ballet, she said, sadly.

"I love them," I told her.

I couldn't wait for mine to get as big as hers. She had to hold them in her hands when we ran to the glass bead store. I fantasized about having to cup my own breasts when I ran.

After Michel and Florence picked me up at the train station, I would skip toward the spacious quiet of Tribeca, euphoric to be reunited with the cement, the metallic smell, the honking yellow cabs, the gum stains, the bums, and the characters who seemed to live out their lives in public.

Michel had my kind of garden—window boxes elevated up over the city, tidy and compact. He kept the loft neat, yet he never complained about housekeeping. He was resourceful, I noticed: rather than use a bed frame, he and Florence had street-picked dozens of tin bunny molds that they used as a platform.

At Michel's loft, I could stare out the windows without worry gnawing at my neck.

One day I saw a girl my age with long blond hair doing trapeze moves on the yellow pipes of the Walk/Don't Walk sign on the street below. I ran down the four flights and joined her. We leaped off stoops and did handstands against the brick buildings. Her name was Justine.

Justine lived with her sister and her mother, Diane, in the loft directly across the street from my father's. Like my mother and

Judy, Diane was also an Unmarried Woman. When Diane was depressed, she would take to her bed, and Justine and I would do the dishes for her because otherwise, they would stay piled up in the big industrial sink they had found on the street. The dishes, it seemed, were troublesome for all the Unmarried Women.

It was always a relief when Diane wasn't home and we didn't have to deal with her needs. Alone with our friends from the neighborhood we could indulge in our romance games, guilt-free. Our games were soap opera versions of playing house and eventually—like a sunflower turns to the sun—we would all end up humping each other in one configuration or another.

"YOUR DOG CURLS UP in your sweater when you're in the city," my mother said with a note of disapproval. I looked at the indifferent dog and found that hard to believe.

"It's too *provincial* here, Mom. They don't understand my humor."

My mother flared her nostrils. She could tell I was working her by using her own line back on her. She often called other people provincial; just recently she had said this about my ballet teacher when I told her that the teacher was planning on playing Dionne Warwick's "I Know I'll Never Love This Way Again" while I did the splits center stage during the next recital.

"You insisted we move here, you wanted the two-story house with your own room, and now you can't *wait* to get out of here," she said.

The more she said it, the more I wanted to get away.

"It's time for *As the World Turns*," I replied, changing the subject.

"Oh my God, you're right, I almost forgot!"

I wanted to kiss the TV.

TV was our unifying force. The soaps brought us together. We started watching *As the World Turns* because a friend of my mother's, Anthony, was on the show. Anthony was the boyfriend of another old friend of my mother's, a cult-horror-movie actress named Barbara Steele, and we used to hang out with both of them in Hollywood. My mother thought it was a riot that he had landed a role playing James Stenbeck, an evil husband to a wife, coincidentally named Barbara. She said Anthony had wanted to be a serious actor, but he couldn't turn down the money.

"Oh, what a riot!" she said as we watched. "Anthony is really believable as a psychopath! Ha ha! Oh, it's so insane, now what is he trying to do—kill her?!"

"I think he's trying to make Barbara think she's going crazy."

"Gaslighting her! Ha! Oh, Alex, it's so funny."

She was happy and entertained; I melted with relief.

IN TRIBECA MY FATHER quietly followed me around the loft with his camera.

He filmed me one evening while I was doing my homework. I had to look up the word *survive* for my class. I free-associated about the word and then I talked to the camera.

I watched the video before I went to bed:

"We will all be famous when I get a lot of money," I said. "I'm gonna buy you and my mom a nice house."

"Everybody eez gonna get a house? You are going to buy me a house when you get rich?" my father asked from behind the camera.

"Yeah, of course."

"I haven't given you very much."

"I don't care. But my mother doesn't want me to give you any money."

"I don't want any money."

"I buy you a nice house. I buy you what you need."

"Alex, you are so cute. You are my best daughter. But I only have one." He laughed.

"That's what I say to my mother," I said. "I say you're my best mother and she says: but you only have one."

"Did you tell your mozer you wanted to give me some money?"

"No, I say, 'When I get older, I'm going to buy you and Michel a house.' She says, 'No, don't give any to your father—he's going to keep taking it and keep taking it . . .'"

Michel laughed.

"The only thing I don't understand is my mother is always screaming at me about you, and it's not about me, it's about you."

"She screamed at you?"

"She wants me to understand, but I don't understand because I love her and I love you. So I don't listen. Sometimes I pretend and I say, *Whaaat?*"

"What do you worry about most?"

"That you guys will get hurt or something. When my mother gets into fights—I worry she'll get hurt . . . and bad stuff will happen. Or that my mother will have to live out on the street. That's what I'm worried about. Or that you guys will have to live out on the street."

ANOTHER EVENING, MICHEL filmed me while I hunched over his desk with Bob's drawing materials and re-created the scenes I loved from the *Penthouse* magazines I found lying around. Porno comics,

I called them. A curvy woman with very precisely drawn fishnet stockings and high heels posing with her ass out. The dialogue in the bubble over her head said: *O yeah, baaaby!* Behind her, a man with a carefully drawn dick pointing toward her round ass; his dialogue bubble said: *Give it to me, baby!* For me, boobs and sex were womanhood, and womanhood was freedom.

"Funny," my father said every now and then in a faraway tone while he was filming me. It was like he was listening almost *too* intently, like the camera had made his senses more acute and more prone to my voice, but also like he had forgotten who I was. He would always return to me, though, and tenderly massage my feet, or slice me impossibly thin pieces of saucisson, handing them to me, one by one, until I could eat no more.

"LET ME WATCH the birth while I eat," I said, referring to the video of myself coming into the world.

That is my scalp, my eyes, my voice crying, I reminded myself while I watched. *That same nose is what sits on my face now, that is me, I came out from inside my mom. That is my mom.*

"This is my favorite part," I mumbled.

"This is good. Your mom yells," he said.

BESIDES THE VIDEOS of myself, Michel only allowed me to watch *The Electric Company, Sesame Street,* and *Saturday Night Live.* He would come in periodically to make sure my thumb wasn't wet from sucking on it (I was supposed to be quitting again) and to make sure I wasn't watching soaps, which he wouldn't let me watch.

I found this surprising because they seemed so innocent compared to *A Coupla White Faggots Sitting Around Talking*—the film he had just made with Gary Indiana. In it, I played the daughter of a dominatrix, although he didn't actually let me watch the scene where Cookie Mueller, who played my mother, pissed on a man and whipped him. But there was a scene where I sat at a bar and smoked a cigar and pretended to drink scotch while chatting with Gary and Taylor Mead. I supposed, for Michel, tacky TV shows were inappropriate, but any kind of art was OK. I didn't agree.

When he went out at night, I'd search public access TV for my true love: *The Robin Byrd Show, Live!* Robin reminded me of Iris, Jodie Foster's street urchin child hooker character in *Taxi Driver*, but only if Iris had become a middle-aged, ragged, soft porn talk show host. Robin hosted the show in a black crocheted bikini, sitting in an all-red room with a neon heart. Here she'd interview naked people. Sometimes they'd suddenly get up from their chair and perform a striptease. I would impatiently wait for the end, which is when they would have an "orgy," but nothing serious ever happened. Still, every episode I was duped into waiting for something more hard-core to unfold.

LATE ONE NIGHT I heard my father and Florence whispering harshly, and then it quickly turned louder. When I opened my door, their bed was dismantled, and Florence was in her underwear throwing the tin bunnies around the room, tits swaying, breathing heavy, skin flushed, her sweat catching the glow from the streetlights, like phosphorescence.

My father laughed that strange, hollow nervous laugh he got

when he was angry, and they chased each other down the hall, behind the green curtain that separated the kitchen and bathroom.

I waited for a while, very still. There was more breathing and struggling. I decided to go to the bathroom to check things out.

They were on the couch near Bob's door, entangled. In the dark, for a moment I thought I was wrong about the fight, and they were actually having sex or play wrestling. But this wasn't like a sexy wrestle in the movies. I stood closer to them trying to decipher the scene.

"It's OK," my father said to me, "go back to bed."

I waited in bed.

Eventually I heard a door slam, and then my father got in bed with me and we cuddled.

"What did I do?" he asked me, crying.

I had never seen him cry before, and while my mother asked me for advice all the time, he never had. Even though I knew it wasn't right to ask me this, I was comforted by the fact that he felt this close to me, this trusting in me.

"Don't worry," I said, squeezing his hand that was draped over my waist. "You didn't do anything."

But I knew he must have done something.

WHATEVER HE HAD done must have been pretty bad because the next thing I knew Florence was in our Essex house, in the kitchen with my mother. I was excited that she was with us, but I suspected this unholy communion wouldn't last.

"All men are alike, Florence!"

My mother was talking to her like she talked to our dog—

impatient with a tad of sympathy but mostly incredulous over the fact that they (the dog and Florence) had not learned their lesson yet.

"They are. All. The. Saaaame!! The bastard-gigolo-junkie bum should be driving a cab to support his family . . ." She paused and from my room I waited for the addendum . . . "But he sure was great to travel with."

Because Florence was staying with us, she cleaned our entire house (as it seemed every guest was required to do), eager to please my mother. The entire time, my mother chastised her cleaning methods with the same dog-training tone.

I stayed out of their way, enjoying the space that my mother's new preoccupation gave me. I loved it when she was fixated on a new person, and I could disappear for a while without worrying.

Eventually, though, I could tell Florence's welcome was beginning to wear thin. I could always feel my mother's intolerance building before anyone else; maybe even before her.

Soon enough, she kicked Florence out and sent her back to Michel. It was a Friday night and I was hoping to be on the train to Grand Central to join Florence in Tribeca the next day.

Saturday morning I was trying to be really sweet and helpful so my mother wouldn't stiffen up when I asked for a ride to the station. She was out in the garden.

"Don't pick any of the baby fennel—OK? It's just getting going," she warned.

I nodded, but the moment she said it, a tender baby stalk appeared in my eyeline. It seemed to call my name. I couldn't resist gently tugging at its roots and feeling it pull free from the silky black soil with that muffled sound like fine hairs ripping from a scalp. I gathered the limp plant in my sweaty palm, soil still clinging to its hairy roots and moved quickly away from the open wound in the ground.

Of course my mother was immediately drawn to the absence. I crushed the baby into my fist and held my fist behind my back.

"Oh my God!!" she screamed, poking at the empty hole.

Panicking, I blamed it on the dog.

"Show me your hand," she demanded.

I stuck out my arm, and she pried open my fist. A little pile of green pulp sat in the center of my palm.

"Absolutely no going to the city this weekend," she said with dead calm and marched me into my room.

I could hear her pacing around the house, aggressively moving things and putting them in different places. I thought if I cried hard enough I could win her sympathies, but her voice outside my door was building, dark and heavy.

"You do whatever you want, traipsing around the city. *You* wanted this dog. You don't give a shit about me. I moved here for *you*. *You* wanted the house with a second story, with the yard. Now all you want to do is get away."

I wept into my pillow. She returned to the familiar rant: "What has your father ever done for you? He didn't contribute a single penny for your eyes. *Not. One. Penny.* He should have gotten a job driving a cab! He's just a damn junkie!"

I wept louder and she said, "Oh, stop exaggerating just so I'll say you can go to the city. That's all you ever think about: When is the first moment you can get out of here, *right*? Well not this time."

I silently vowed to never forgive her. I didn't know who she was anymore. She was cruel, inhuman, maybe even possessed by the devil.

In a couple of hours, though, she came into my room and sat on the bed.

"I overreacted," she admitted.

She cuddled me and told me how much she loved me, and everything that was good about us came rushing back. I apologized as well. I was so sorry for lying about the baby fennel, about wanting to go to my dad's.

"I didn't want to go to the city anyway," I told her as we cleaned the kitchen together later.

It was strange, but I could barely remember why I had been so mad earlier.

After we cleaned, we went out to see the stars. It was a beautiful summer night, very dark and humid with fireflies lighting up the yard like hundreds of full moons. She prepared glass bottles with perforated aluminum foil tops to house the live fireflies. We set out into the garden with these homemade traps.

Back inside with our treasures, we turned off all the lights, placed the jars of fireflies on the bedroom windowsill, and snuggled under the covers.

As I fell asleep, there were moments of blackness, when no fireflies were lit, and then suddenly the whole room glowed, casting smoky shadows on the ceiling that would be scary if we hadn't been under the covers together. Sometimes the flies maintained a rhythm, pulsing the dark room like soft yellow strobes.

Late in the night I heard my mother getting up and opening the windows. I watched her sleepily let the fireflies go free so they wouldn't die in the jars.

Now

I'm nervously preparing the house. For the first time, everyone is coming to Philadelphia for Christmas: my stepmom, Cindy; my sister, Gaby, and her family; and Viva, who's still camping out in Miko's room (and he is thrilled he gets to sleep with us in the big bed, every night, while she's here).

I want the house to be cozy and inviting. I want the kids to sense no tension. I want warmth and ease, free-flowing conversation. Still, as I prepare for the visitors, I am making the mental list of what can't be said in my mother's earshot (within a square mile), and what can't be suggested either, through gesture or word.

Currently, Viva is trying to "help" me clean as she marches around the house, gossiping with her sister Marybeth, in between going on about the light: our house does not have enough of it (I agree but won't admit it), but then again, according to her, it's too light at night; at night we need more of the dark.

"You need a maid," she says.

"Housekeeper," I correct.

I can feel her roll her eyes behind my back.

She is wearing layers of long bedclothes and Uggs, and her hair is still blond and frizzy. Her blue eyes have suffered from typical old age afflictions like dryness and floaters and films and a slight separation of the rim of the lower lid from the eyeball, which becomes irritated and reddened.

She paces around, phone in hand, looking for something—the eternal search for a number written on a scrap of paper—while she asks Marybeth about the lawsuit.

It seems like the siblings have been suing one another for years, so it's hard to keep track of who is on whose side at the moment. I'm not sure if it's just my mother, or my mother is suing all of them, or if one group of siblings has banded together to sue another group.

"I mean can you believe the hideous thing Terry built? That piece of land has the best light. And it has the only good view. Mm-hmm. Unbelievable. What a pig. I never, never should have sold it. Well, now Chrissy's derelict kids have usurped the little bay, so it's no use . . ."

Grandma died from Alzheimer's when I was in college, and Grandpa died on his birthday in 2005—that's when the fighting and the lawsuits over the house and land started.

When the house was finally sold—against the wishes of some of the siblings—the family kept a large chunk of property across the bay that extends all the way to the bridge. They parceled it out among the nine siblings, but the disagreements over who got what piece of land have never ended.

Marybeth was "*Fucking* Marybeth" for a long time, but she seems to be Viva's ally at the moment.

After the call with Marybeth, my mother yells to me, "Honey, this house is so dark! You've got it all wrong. At night you can't have any light! I'll send you the article. Not the blue light from the computers, but also not the streetlight. Lui has to have blackout curtains. I'll buy them for you."

She has some money from finally selling off her parcel of land to a sibling, I think, but my sister, Gaby, pays for the majority of her expenses, so when she says, "I'll buy something or other for you," it's suspect.

"But right now let's clean these living room windows and get some more light in this room. Because you have to get vitamin D from the sun! Did you come into this house, in the daytime, before you bought this house? Probably not. God, they are absolutely filthy! Nick! When is the last time you cleaned these windows?"

"Yeah, Nick," I say, shooting my husband a conspiratorial glance. "When did you last clean these windows?"

"I was waiting for you to arrive, Viva, so we could work on them together."

My mother rolls her eyes and says, "OK, Nick, I'll do it."

She thinks he is trying to get out of it, or to somehow manipulate the situation so she ends up cleaning the widows by herself. The truth is he really gets a kick out of her. But she decided, awhile back, that he was a "liar." He's a filmmaker, so over the years he has tried—or really, *we* have tried—to capture her. It's a great way to spend time with her—filming what's going on, interviewing her, documenting the state of things—it provides a buffer. We made a short film about her preparing for a painting show she had at a gallery in Santa Barbara, and about fifteen years ago we started a larger project documenting a gig she had in a new film Paul Morrissey was making. That project was left unfinished and ended badly. Somewhere along the way she decided Nick was exploiting her—like Michel, she said, and like Andy too, and like all the men in her life.

As she cleans the windows, still talking about blackout curtains, I hang the Christmas lights, imagining myself like a turtle in winter, sliding deep down under the thick layers of ice, waiting with shallow breath, so still, eyes open, but heart slowed down to a barely perceptible beat.

Chapter 9

The River

coached my mother along the drive. We were going to the River while we searched for a new place to live again. We had to leave the Essex house after Chamberlain had fired her—or she had quit—depending on how she told the story.

"Stay calm," I said. "Remember: What do you care what they do? They're idiots. Just smile and nod your head."

"OK, honey, thanks."

"Promise?"

"I promise, really. You are so smart."

"Smile and nod your head."

I believed that if I stayed physically close to her at the River, I could stop a fight, like the one that happened a few years ago. But I knew when she was alone, anything could happen.

I scanned the horizon for the peaks of the green suspension bridge.

"I see the bridge!" I yelled.

Soon we were on the bridge, heading toward Wellesley Island, the wide blue river ribboning out on either side; I could see our tiny dock and the 210 channel marker at the tip of our little peninsula, and then we were crunching down the gravel driveway, and the big house appeared.

As we approached the house, my mother was frantic, worried one of her sisters had "stolen" her favorite bedroom. It used to be her grandmother's room, she said, before she was carted off to the loony bin. She liked its large bay windows with *good light,* its blue flower wallpaper, the fact that it was on the opposite end of the hall from Grandma and Grandpa's room, and that it had less motorboat noise than the other bedrooms.

Luckily for us it was empty, and so we claimed it for ourselves.

"Amazing that none of them have swiped this room already," she said while she shoved all the windows open.

Closed windows infuriated her.

THAT SUMMER I STAYED CLOSE with my cousin Steve and his younger sister, Franny. We were a threesome, though only Steve and I sometimes tried kissing.

Steve had just turned ten, and was so handsome, I thought, with his shiny blond hair and freckles. I was still nine, and I wanted to impress him. I wanted to kiss him like the women on *As the World Turns*—smooth and graceful, pressing our mouths deeply into each other with husky, sure voices, heads falling from side to side like a pretty dance.

The reality was our teeth clicked together, and it was more analytical than I had imagined.

In France you could marry your cousin. Marybeth had always suggested I marry her son, Oliver, which annoyed me because he was such a baby. But Steve seemed mature. I had a bad crush on him, and anytime he went off to play golf or tennis with the aunts and uncles, it hurt. I wished the sports would go to hell.

One morning when Steve was cheating on me with golf, I overheard Chrissy and her husband, John, having sex. I persuaded Franny to hide with me in the adjoining closet so we could spy on them. I knew Franny was too young to see such a thing, but I couldn't help myself.

"Oh yes, yes, John, honey," Chrissy was moaning.

I slid down underneath a long coat and tried to get a better view of the action. Franny crouched next to me.

"Don't speak," I whispered to her.

"Harder, Christine, harder," John said.

"What are they doing?" Franny asked.

I silently mouthed the word: *fucking*. Franny opened her eyes wide, and I motioned for her to look through the crack in the door. Aunt Chrissy was lying on her side, her pregnant belly jutting forward with a rhythmic motion, the sheets tangled around her legs. John's hairy hands were gripping her hips. We couldn't see their faces.

Chrissy called out in a breathy high voice, "I'm coming, honey, yes, oh . . ."

"What's coming?" Franny asked, confused. "What's happening?"

I put my finger to my lips and we both waited. Silence and then rustling sheets. A door opening and water running. We scrambled out of the closet and ran down the hall giggling.

"I told you a long time ago," I said impatiently. "That's how a baby is made."

I was satisfied with how shocked Franny looked. I wanted to

corrupt her in some way, to show her the ways of the world because her innocence annoyed me. I blamed her mother for it. My mother had said that her sisters were all "naive and petite bourgeoisie," the meaning of which I wasn't quite sure, but it seemed that not knowing how sex worked at Franny's age was a symptom.

IT WAS HARD to tell whether my mother was loved or loathed by the family. My aunts seemed to want her attention and, at times, all six of them would gossip and laugh as though they were the best of friends. Then, unexpectedly, things could change. She might say something to make them mad, like how putting perfume on babies was "so petit bourgeois," and when she left the room they would speak Franglais.

"Absolutely fou, la mère, non?" Marybeth might say.

"Arête, arête, it doesn't matter," Chrissy would defend, gesturing toward me. "Elle comprend tout."

I'm not an idiot, I thought about yelling at them. *I know what you are saying.*

After, I'd join my mother and report back to her about what the aunts were saying, doing an imitation of them so she would know I wasn't totally seduced by them.

"We've gooooot to get the kids into actiiiiivities! They've goooot to get up and out! Oooh my vagiiiina is aaaaching!" I would say in my best Marybeth impression.

"Ha ha!" she said. "Alex, we've got to get you on *Saturday Night Live*! You are *so* funny!"

"Mom, they don't have kids on the show."

"Well, you can be the first one, honey. You are better than any of those adults. I'm going to call Lorne."

————

ONE LAZY AFTERNOON Steve and I sat in the yellow raft, floating in the cattail marsh beyond the boathouse. From there I could see my mother painting at her easel, which she had set up on the strip of dock behind the boathouse. She was in a big straw hat with a sarong draped over the brim and white zinc oxide on her nose. For her, getting a sunburn was worse than being drawn and quartered.

Of course she couldn't just be happy painting. She had to find something to get mad about. From that location she could see the end of the main dock and would periodically yell at the little boy cousins about how they were juvenile delinquents or that they were going to drown or hook an eyeball out with the fishing rods. I found it annoying the way she would get into the cousins' business—if my aunts didn't care what their own kids were doing, why should she?

A glint of silver in the sky caught our attention. My mother looked up, shading her eyes from the sun. A small plane swooped low, and the sound of the engine drifted off as it headed toward the landing strip in Watertown. The aunts at the end of the dock started jumping up and down waving to the sky.

"Bob's here," my mother said with a doomy tone.

"*Uncle* Bob you mean," I yelled from the raft, making a gagging face.

Steve laughed.

After Bob arrived, I made sure to keep my distance. He and my mother were inseparable, though. They talked about the cosmos, and poems, and some American Indian thing where you swallow the beating heart of a fish to get more life force into your own body.

One morning they actually went fishing, brought the live fish up to the fish-gutting porch, sliced it open and pulled out its beating heart. My mother massaged the heart in the palm of her hand to keep it beating and slipped the dark red glob into her mouth and swallowed it whole. Bob seemed incredibly impressed.

I almost vomited.

A FEW NIGHTS LATER, at dinner, I could tell my mother was in a mood. Maybe the beating fish heart gave her too much "life force," maybe Bob's presence unnerved her, maybe one of her sisters had said something to set her off, but I could sense something building, gathering around her edges.

My aunts dimmed the lights, and Chrissy lit all the candles in the big ceramic grapevine candelabra at the center of the table.

My mother rolled her eyes.

Grandpa complained that he couldn't see anything while Jeannie served him at the head of the table, cutting his meat for him.

"Have some kale, Dad," my mother said.

"Too many damn vegetables," Grandpa replied, and then baby talked to Jeannie. "Just lovely sweetheart, yes, yes," he said, caressing Jeannie's back while she fiddled with his plate.

"Pathetic," my mother mumbled.

Jeannie whispered in his ear, "You don't have to eat what Sue cooked, Dad."

"Yeah, Dad," my mother said. "We don't give a shit if you croak. Ha ha!"

I nudged her.

While all this was going on, some invisible force was making Bob arrange all the stuff around him into symmetrical patterns, as if he had secret orders in his head about how things had to go together. As he spoke, he moved his hands slowly and deliberately so that eventually he had a neat little barrier around his plate made from the corn on the cob holders, his silverware, two wineglasses, a napkin, and the three crystal teardrops from the broken chandelier above the table.

"Is your father still so damn handsome?" Chrissy asked me.

I tried to think of something that would make everyone laugh. "He sleeps naked in a silk scarf!"

"God, he was just so adorable with those tight pants and long hair."

Right then, Grandpa asked me to check if Mary's lights were turned on. I was relieved to get outside for a couple of minutes. I walked to the edge of the porch stairs and looked out toward Mary's hill. The flagpoles were clanking in the wind. I couldn't see her, but the lights at her feet were reflected in the mist and made a light halo above her head. I went back inside to tell Grandpa they were working.

Something had happened.

I should never have left her alone.

Grandpa was standing up at the end of the table, yelling. "None of you girls ever ran away! Why would you? Enjoyed yourselves just as much under your own roof! Crazy Sue, putting those ideas into their heads. Trouble starter. Nothing but trouble. Never made a penny."

"Oh, just *forget* it," my mother yelled. "I mean, Jesus! I just wanted a loan—a thousand or so, until Alex and I settle down into another house."

I quickly sat down next to my mother and took her hand into mine and whispered, "Remember? Can't you remember? Just smile."

Her hand was cold and stiff. She shook her head yes as though she were listening to me, and she smiled like she was locked in a box, and she just kept on talking and glaring at Grandpa with her shark eyes.

Bob addressed the table as he tidied a barrier of silverware: "It's very interesting what the mind chooses to remember; some say the left hemisphere of the—"

My mother interrupted with an "Oh! Oh! Oh!" and everyone looked at her, pretending they were startled. She tried to stand up, but I held her down. "Dad doesn't remember *anything*, Bob. Neither does Mom, neither does Jeannie, neither does John, neither does anyone—it's incredible. Their left hemispheres are all screwed up. Dad says he never hit Johnny or me."

I squeezed her leg and narrowed my eyes, but she continued anyway. "John had to hide in the school bathroom because Dad beat him so badly. Mom, don't you remember when Dad broke your ribs?"

Grandma stood up and pointed at my mother. "It's all in your imagination!"

Barb said, "Why don't we think of more pleasant things?"

Jeannie pulled on my mother's sleeve and used her angry voice. "What's wrong with you?" she hissed. "You're really upsetting Mom now."

Grandma pointed at my mother again and said, almost out of breath, "You're always, *always* starting things!"

My mother took a deep breath and began a monologue. The first couple of lines were delivered casually, but as she continued, her voice began to rise with the veins in her neck.

"Well, Dad, can you blame me for actually taking care of my only daughter? I mean let's thank God I'm not one of those mothers who let the nanny raise the children! *Or* who let them cry all day and night in their cribs—let alone even own a crib like all your *other* pathetic bourgeois daughters do—but just you wait and see when *their* kids grow up to be serial killers. All I want is a *paltry* thousand fucking dollars to buy some Moon Boots and a down coat for my daughter, who may freeze and starve this winter, and you're attacking *me*? *Me*?!"

"Where do you get all your crazy ideas from?" Grandpa asked. "Why bother coming over at all if you're just going to be trouble? Having sex . . . darn it all! Gallivanting with no husband . . ."

"And that book . . . full of *smut*," Grandma added.

"Now let's calm down," Chrissy said. "We all know that Sue has a wild imagination, and who cares what happened years ago or whatever anyway? Let's just eat our pie and enjoy the night."

"It's better for your health, Sue, if you *control* your anger," another aunt piped up.

"I'm not angry," my mother said. "I'm just saying that it's hard not to be perfect like everyone else. I wish I had a rich husband waiting on me hand and foot and attending to my every whim and whose cock Dad practically sucks because he loves all men so much. I've always suspected he had an affair with his old assistant Ed Reilly."

I knew when she said "cock" it was over.

Grandpa stood up. His voice was weaving in and out of clarity. "Don't you ever touch a curtain . . . That filthy book of yours! You'll never amount to anything with that nose of yours!"

A few of my aunts joined him. Their voices turned both hoarse and shrill, their faces contorted.

"Look at you, you filthy bag lady! You're the nympho in your movies!"

"You make me sick, Sue, get out of here!"

"You ruin everything, *everything*!"

My mother stood up and gripped the table so hard her knuckles turned a bright shocking white. The veins popped in her temples. I wrapped myself around her waist, hoping she would come to, recognize me, and calm down. Under my arms I could feel her muscles quiver and go hard under her skin.

"Every single one of you at this table is a liar!" she said with a dark, rumbling voice.

Grandma walked over and placed her hands on my mother's shoulders, directly above my head. She started to shake my mother and repeat: "You always lie. Always. Lie, lie, lie."

Please, please, I prayed.

Grandpa stood up, leaned forward, closed his eyes, and pounded his fists on the table. "Filthy whore good-for-nothing!" he yelled.

"You tell her, Dad!" Jeannie cheered.

I felt myself rise up, still attached like an urchin to my mother's torso as she reached over the center of the table and grabbed the huge candelabra, flames dancing. She paused for a moment, or time stopped, drips of hot wax landed on my face, and then she threw it, and it went flying across the room in an arc, all the little flames flickering out as it whipped past Grandpa's head and smashed into the mirror above the sideboard, cracking it down the center.

The room was dark and still. Calm, even.

Then a figure was moving through the dark space, something black and lumbering.

Grandpa.

He was sputtering about the candelabra coming from Germany. The table was vibrating.

Frisbees were suddenly flying through the air, one after another, smashing against things, sending white shards back, and I realized that my mother was throwing plates.

I was lifted off my feet and dragged away by my neck, backward, through the shrapnel.

I tried to wriggle free so I could save my mother. I twisted myself so I could see who had snatched me: Marybeth.

As she dragged me past the piano, I saw that Grandpa was on my mother, and they both went toppling over onto the floor.

Marybeth clasped her hand over my eyes as she dragged, but I could still see between her fingers, like the balusters of the stair banister. I saw figures sitting at the table watching while Grandpa pinned my mother down to the floor, knelt on top of her, and started beating her, blood splattering upward—little sprays in the dark.

As Marybeth continued to drag me, she hissed in my ear, "This is all your mother's fault."

Suddenly, through the jumble of bodies and pounding feet, my mother was reaching for me, pulling me away from Marybeth. We were intertwined again, running in slow motion toward the front door. I could feel the family closing in around us.

As my mother struggled with the doorknob, Grandma slumped into a chair right next to the door. My face was almost touching her sticky-stiff curls, bleached and dyed like pale-pink cotton candy on the top of her head. I took a fistful of it and yanked, but the motion came out feebly.

We leaped down the front stairs, past the reindeer, moving furtively across the lawn, our gasps making little breathy ghosts dance in the cool air.

In the moonlight I could see that bright blood, almost fluorescent, had soaked my mother's white clothes. I felt woozy and held on to her.

This is it, I thought, *she's about to die.*

I heard my own scratchy voice coming out, asking her about the head wound I assumed she had. I heard her telling me that it was actually Grandpa's blood all over her sweat suit, not her own, but that her big toe was cut deeply and she was afraid it might be about to fall off.

She can survive a missing toe, I thought. Then I imagined the dark slash at the base of the big toe, the toe dangling off the foot by a thread of dark tendon, glistening bone gristle.

We finally got to the cabin door. It slammed shut behind us and we called 911. We huddled on the floor by the phone and waited until the walls turned red from the ambulance lights.

Two ambulances arrived at the same time.

When we limped out of the cabin, I could see Grandpa and Jeannie across the lawn, standing at the top of the big house's front stairs. Grandpa had a white towel wrapped around his forearm, and Jeannie held him by the good arm. Even from that far I could see the red soaking through the towel. They seemed to be just waiting at the top of the stairs, shell-shocked, standing in the dark like two zombies. We looked at them, looking out at *us*.

I understood that we were now mortal enemies. My mother and me, a couple of lone survivors on the other side of the lawn.

But then another feeling washed over me. It was more familiar. I wanted to yell out, "Hey, Grandpa, Jeannie—see you at the hospital!"

Maybe we were comrades, after all.

MY MOTHER WAS SILENT in her emergency room bed, separated from Grandpa only by a thick green plastic curtain. Her right big toe was sewn up at the base with twelve stitches. The inner part of Grandpa's forearm got thirty-six stitches in all.

In the waiting room Chrissy and Jeannie stared at me with

pained eyes. I could have easily curled up in their laps, sucking my thumb, if only I could have been sure they wouldn't say anything bad about my mother. I didn't want to hear one more bad thing. I knew from their sorry gazes that they thought I was sticking with my mother just because I had to. I tried to be still and neutral, tried to go down deep for a while and wait it out, suck my thumb down there, and let everyone do their thing on the surface.

I wondered if we could ever go back to the house again after this.

Jeannie broke the silence: "You know, honey, all this is really your mother's fault—*she* started it."

If I'd had the stretch of lawn between us again, I would have told her that I hated her and to fuck off, or that it was all her own fascist fault, but this close? I still wanted them to think I was sweet.

She wouldn't drop it, though. "You do know that, don't you, darling?" she prodded. "That it was your mother's fault?"

It made me so sick to do it, but I nodded my head.

Yes.

Part 2

THE CHELSEA

1980–1985

Chapter 10

The State of Things

We stood under the red and white–striped awning like two dusty travelers who had just left their horses at the corral and were ready for a warm bed.

I had watched myself in Michel's videos toddling on the sidewalk under this very same striped awning with the numbers 222, but those videos were in black and white. This felt like Dorothy stepping into Technicolor Oz. I was standing in the shadow of the real ten-story brick building. It was as full of breath and as raw as quaking bodies. Above me bluish-white neon letters ran vertically down the center of the building like a vein spelling the word: HOTEL. Below the vein, much smaller red neon letters ran perpendicularly, glowing like a heart beating out the word: CHELSEA. At the entrance I stared at the Dylan Thomas bronze plaque. *Sid* was scrawled across the bottom in black spray paint.

"Who's Sid?" I asked my mother.

"An asshole rock star who stabbed his girlfriend on the first floor, and everyone's obsessed with him."

We pushed open the heavy glass doors and stepped into the lobby.

"She's back!" Jerry cheered from the front desk.

There he was, the same bald desk clerk who had been there while my mother was in labor with me on this very same red carpet. Behind him was the wall of mail-and-key cubbies—a box for each room. I remembered these, or maybe I had seen them in the videos.

We are about to get our own box, I told myself.

We walked forward along the dark red carpet, and I compared reality to Michel's videos. There was the large fireplace with its ornate wood mantelpiece, there were the two vinyl benches—*they are bright red!*—with carved wooden armrests. There were the benches with black-and-white padded vinyl tops—*actually black-and-white!*—and mirrored bases. I draped myself over one of them, basking in the vibe.

Above me a big papier-mâché lady, painted white, sat on a swing hanging from the ceiling. Across from me a large painting of upside-down rainbows on black shelves. Also, one of a man wearing a hat, his face exploding with squirts of paint. My mother said all the lobby art was "hideous."

"The first Chelsea baby has returned!" a slim man in a gray suit said as he stepped out of an office to the side of the lobby. Smoke seemed to billow from behind him as he reached out to me. I was happy to be recognized. He said, "Look at you! I don't know how you survived your crazy parents." I bristled but hugged him anyway.

Apparently, we owed Stanley, this gray-suited man, loads of money from "the old days," but he still let us move back in. He gave some tenants cheap deals in exchange for art and/or publicity.

"You need me," my mother was telling him. "I'm good publicity because I'm the only one left from the old days since Andy made all the money."

We piled our bags on Jerome-the-bellman's cart and followed Stanley. He led us into a gold elevator. People had scratched all sorts of things into the gold paint. There was *Sid* again, scratched in next to the buttons.

As the numbers above the doors lit up, Jerome sighed.

The elevator stopped.

The third floor? My heart sank.

I could feel my mother getting agitated. I knew she hated the lower floors—no good light.

"At least it's in the back," I whispered to my mother as we exited the gold elevator, our footsteps echoing in the marble hall.

Stanley unlocked the door and presented the single room like it was a suite in the Plaza.

"This tiny thing?" my mother said as he handed her the key. "Jesus."

I looked at Jerome. He was slim, black, and wore a loose brown suit. He shrugged. I smiled. I wanted him to like me, but I suspected he couldn't care less.

"When you can afford more, let me know, Viva," Stanley said. "We have a one-bedroom on the seventh floor opening up soon."

WE SETTLED INTO THIS not-right room for a bit, tried our best to accept the bad light, the mustard-colored upholstery, and the shaggy rug that smelled like cigarette smoke. The view was a solid wall of buildings on Twenty-second Street. Even I felt we were destined for something better than this.

I waited while our enemy Ronald Reagan was trying to get rid of our love Jimmy Carter; John Lennon got shot and we swayed with a sea of crying people outside the Dakota; Yoko Ono stood on the balcony, a tiny figure clad in black, yellow cabs honking when they passed.

I was reenrolled at PS 3.

Meanwhile, my mother had a regular column in the Style Section of *The Village Voice*. She had just published an article about how hard it was to find a good couch, and she was working on one about how to dress your children for under ten dollars. Zoe and I modeled the outfits, and my mother took the pictures of us posing in the lobby wearing flannel nightgowns from Lamstons and earrings we had made from feathers at the fish and tackle store a couple of doors down.

All of this felt right and good; we were in the center of things; the rhythm of NYC was in my bones.

Although plenty of people came through the Chelsea, and we quickly made friends with many of the permanent residents, the Chelsea felt like mine.

The interior was all gray marble. The grand stairwell ran down the center of the building and split it in half—each floor's landing had two elevators and swinging doors that led to the main halls on either side, with smaller hall tributaries that branched off.

Along the halls were brown doors with brass knockers, and behind them were apartments: empty apartments, apartments with people passing through, and apartments with long-term residents who decorated their space so thoroughly that the interior bled out from the seams of their doors and into the hallways—turquoise paint, gold enamel, plants, stickers, and plastic toys. Voices and music could be heard from behind the brown doors. Crying and fighting too.

Things quickly turned sour between my mother and Stanley, so I had to learn to navigate a sometimes hostile landscape and, by listening for the creak of Stanley's office doors, how to avoid being harangued for rent when I passed through the lobby.

But still, I prided myself on how I fit in there, how I knew every nook and secret spot of the hotel.

Occasionally, when I left the apartment, I would grab a Barbie doll on my way out. Before I went wherever I was going, I would unlatch a little hatch door on a pipe that was nestled in the corner of the stairwell and ran the length of the building. We called it the key shoot.

I'd rip off the Barbie head and drop it into the pipe and wait until I heard a faint thud when it landed in a little latched glass window behind the operator's booth. (Sometimes the new operator would lean out from the booth, dangling the head from its hair, and say, "This yours?" and I would act like I had no idea what she was talking about.)

Occasionally when I was in the lobby, I might lift the red vinyl seat of one of the chairs and climb inside it, closing the lid and performing this disappearing act for tourists. I would lie still in my dark coffin for a bit, imagining what the tourists were doing.

She's glancing down at her own seat and wondering if hers opens like a coffin as well. He's squashing out his cigarette in the tin top of the tall black ashtray.

When I climbed back out again, the tourist always smiled at me. I smiled back and was tempted to pull the St. Pauli Girl from the brown paper bag I had just bought for my mother at the Middle Deli to show the tourist how kids in NYC could buy beer for their parents.

I would call out to Jerry in a very loud, familiar way—*"Hey,*

Jerry! Any mail?"—and poke my head around the partition to search the wall of boxes. I knew we had no mail; I was just hoping a tourist might be watching.

Then I would slip into the operator's booth to grab a quick hug from Josephine, who had also been there when I was born. She had snow-white hair and a body like the papier-mâché swing lady. She would pull me to her big bosom, where I would disappear for a few seconds while she controlled the old-fashioned operator's board.

"*ChelseaHotelmayIhelp* you?" Her light and airy voice sounded muffled with my face buried in her bosom.

Two elevators faced the front desk, green and gold.

I always avoided the green—it was dreary.

Beyond the gold elevator were the secret back doors to the El Quijote. Behind those doors lived the dark guts of the Spanish restaurant that most people entered from the sidewalk. I would sometimes sneak into the restaurant to pee or tend to my recurring bloody noses in the sink of the Chiquita bathroom with the flamenco lady dancing on the door.

I loved the salty dank smell of boiled lobster that greeted me before my eyes adjusted to the dark restaurant, where each red banquette had its own little red glowing lamp; the white-aproned waiters floated around in that red underworld, holding silver trays with steaming baked potatoes and piles of mussels; and the cozy bar served sad drunks who had been sitting since the middle of the day. I wondered if maybe they didn't know they had been there all day because it always seemed like the same time in there.

When I wasn't at the Chelsea, I was at the Squat.

I had discovered it one weekend while I was at my father's loft, and he took me on an errand. We arrived at a narrow building that looked like an old Italian villa with two cute iron balconies on the second floor. Above a tall and wide storefront window was a large hand-painted silver sign that said Squat Theatre in red letters.

It was only halfway down the block from the Chelsea but in another world altogether—four stories of dark-humored, hairy, affectionate Hungarian immigrants and a gaggle of their kids. One of the kids, Rebecca, called Rebi, would soon become my dearest friend. We began to ride the school bus home together from PS 3.

Between the Chelsea and the Squat I was free and happy; it felt like I had finally found a place to call home.

I BLEW OUT TEN CANDLES on February 21 on a movie set in Lisbon.

The movie was called *The State of Things,* and in it my mother played the script girl and I played her daughter, Alexandra. It was a movie about making a movie. The story is that the producers of the movie within the movie—a sci-fi—run out of money and the cast and crew have to bide their time in an empty hotel by the sea.

In it, the script girl (my mother) is having a passionate affair with the director of the sci-fi, played by the actor Patrick Bauchau, aka "the Wet Kisser."

When I first started calling him the Wet Kisser, my mother howled with laughter. I assumed she was laughing because she was in agreement with my assessment—that he was a slimy-lipped lothario trying to pull the wool over her eyes, but I was worried she seemed to have a type. There were distinct similarities between Bob Fulton and Patrick Bauchau. I was willing to admit that they both had an elegance about them with their floppy side-parted hair falling over an eye, their lanky height, and their understated confidence, but I knew they were smarmy and pretentious under their rumpled linen blazers.

The director, Wim Wenders, also wore rumpled linen blazers and had similar features to the other men—the long lanky limbs, the same deep creases around his lips and eyes—but the difference was, well . . . I loved him. He was generous and straightforward. He respected Camilla and me (Camilla played the Wet Kisser's daughter), and he told us what he needed for each scene with tenderness. As long as we hit our marks, he let us make up our own lines. He filmed us sitting in an abandoned car on the side of an ocean cliff while we talked about life and death.

I would have welcomed Wim as my mother's boyfriend. I sensed they had a flirtation going on—or at least I sensed that my mother was attracted to him, which made it even more frustrating when I later found out that she was indeed having an affair with the Wet Kisser.

The day I discovered it, we were filming. Camilla's and my characters were supposed to be listening through the door while the script girl and the director had sex in the adjoining room.

When it was time to film the real sex scene, the set was closed, but Camilla and I snuck in and peeked at the action through the gaps between bodies and equipment. In a pool of red lighting, I saw my mother's frizzy hair, her slight body draped in nothing but an oversize man's shirt, writhing atop the Wet Kisser, arching her spine. It felt familiar—she was doing her vibrating-breathing-Muktananda-meditation hand gestures—touching the tip of her middle finger and tip of her thumb together while raising her arms above her head. My stomach dropped.

She's good, I thought. *Too good.*

I was suspicious.

Does she really want to have sex with the Wet Kisser, or is she just acting? Or is she actually really having sex?

Camilla was titillated; I pretended to be, but it disgusted me. For Camilla's sake, I also pretended to be disappointed when we were discovered spying and kicked off the set. Camilla wanted to know more, but I had seen enough.

AWHILE BACK I had made up my own origin story that my mother loved and always asked me to repeat. The story was simple: from heaven I examined all the potential parents in the world until I finally found Vivah Supahstahhhh, and I implanted myself in her womb. The idea being that not only were we destined to be together but that I voluntarily chose her because she was exceptional. I made it up because I knew it would please her, but she seemed to take it literally. She said the story made sense because when I was four, she took a little acid with some friends on the River and I walked up to her holding a little piece of tinfoil with two baby teeth marks on it. There was acid inside the folded tinfoil, she said, but she couldn't be sure I had ingested any.

Instead of taking me to a hospital, where she feared they would pump my stomach, she took me out on the boat, to the calm river, and when she looked into my big eyes, she saw the whole universe swirling in my pupils. She believed I was God.

"What did I do?" I asked her.

"You laughed a lot."

I couldn't remember this, but I always pictured it—our hair blowing in the wind, the slate river zooming past us, my laughter, her blue eyes looking into mine where the cosmos swirled around.

She must have told Wim about all this because he asked me to tell my origin story in the movie. The fact that he wanted our family mythology to be in his movie gave me a deep sense that our life was magical and infused with purpose, though I was unsure what our purpose was. *Maybe*, I thought, *it was just to delight and entertain others with our charm and humor.*

It was with this mindset that I felt emboldened to pray for a baby sister when we visited the statue of Our Lady of Fatima in Sintra. My mother had always loved these religious icons and sites of religious pilgrimages.

Why not add to our clan? The baby would be meant for us, a magical child, a boon for the world.

During our pilgrimage to Fatima, I worked myself up into what I felt was a deep mystical state and whispered my wish to a penny—*please, a baby sister*—and threw the coin into the water at her feet.

A month after we arrived home from Portugal, I found my mother moaning on the bed in our room. When I asked her what was wrong, she blurted out: "Oh, honey! I'm pregnant!" I jumped up and down with excitement, somersaulted on the bed, then threw myself to the floor in ecstasy.

"Should I have an abortion?" she asked.

What? Kill our miracle?! Fatima had granted my wish! An abortion was the most ridiculous suggestion I had ever heard. I would not even entertain the idea of aborting our baby.

"But we have no money," she sighed, "and we live on a postage stamp of an apartment . . . and there's no father . . ."

A father? Jesus. I had never considered a father. When I prayed at Fatima, I hadn't thought about the sex part of having a baby. I wanted an immaculate conception. I had imagined that her pregnancy was a direct result of my desire, not *sexual* desire. I wanted a sidekick to collaborate with, someone alongside me who would be able to share and witness the ineffable life we were living.

I stood in the middle of the living room suddenly gripped with dread.

Please, no.

"The Wet Kisser?!" I asked in horror.

My mother shook her head: *no.*

Then who the hell is the father? We are together all the time. How is this possible?

"It's Anthony," she finally said, sighing again. "And he wants nothing to do with the baby."

Anthony? Our old soap opera actor friend? I had to get my bearings to get over the shock of realizing that since we had gotten back from Portugal she'd had actual secret sex with Anthony.

I forced myself to quickly recover because I didn't want her to think she had made any mistakes or leave any room for doubt. It was up to me to make sure we kept this baby.

"Who cares?" I said boldly, hugging her, dismissing the fact that she had chosen a man who was playing a nefarious master manipulator, and an eventual murdering psychopath. "Who cares as long as we have a little girl. That's what I asked at Fatima."

"Me too," my mother admitted.

I must have been siphoning her internal monologue, my psyche living inside her body like a growth on an organ when I'd prayed for the same thing.

"Now we can get the bigger apartment," I reminded her.

Now

Viva's on the phone again, still following me around the house. I have no idea whom she's talking to, but she'll probably try to put me on the phone with them soon.

Gaby and her family will be arriving any moment.

"You didn't know? Alex is a famous yoga teacher now. Uh-huh, and she had two kids! No, but she begged for her mommy during Lui's birth! *Ha ha!*"

In the tone of her laugh there is both mockery and a kind of wicked thrill over the irony of it. The irony being, according to her, that even though I didn't invite her to my home birth, I still called her name.

"It's true," I say, as I pass her. "I did call out for you."

My mother is still holding the phone to her ear, responding to the other person on the line with "Ha!" and "Uh-huh" and You're kidding" when she nears the shelf with the photo albums.

This puts me on edge; I would prefer to keep our wedding and birth albums secreted away from her. Seeing the photos might trigger a wicked mood.

While she was visiting for the wedding, we had prepared for the worst by asking a mutual friend to be her "handler" in case she needed to be physically removed from our house, which she did when she found out that

Michel had been living, for years, right around the corner from us. His house was hard to miss—he was famous in the neighborhood for letting his lawn grow into a wild field and then mowing spiral jetty-like paths through it, and he was often on his porch, bird-watching in his sarong—and we had gone to great lengths to hide this from her. But eventually she discovered our secret, and it threw her into a dark and brooding mood culminating in a twisted wedding toast that had some advice on how you should pray for sons rather than daughters and concluding with her throwing books down our stairs that she suspected we had stolen from her storage unit. That's when the friend had to usher her out.

And then, a year later, I didn't invite her to Lui's birth.

I am now trying to remember if my father is in any of the birth photos in the album. We had invited him and his girlfriend over right after I birthed the placenta. I never told my mother he visited that night. Even though it was fifteen years ago, knowing he was there could send her into a three-day rage.

When I got pregnant with Lui, I never considered anything other than a water birth at home. Our house then was a cute old clapboard farmhouse near Hudson, New York. When word got around that the local yoga teacher was having a home birth, the phone rang. It was our neighbors—two lovely older gay men (one had been a well-known obstetrician)—calling to tell me that what I was planning was really dangerous and begging me to reconsider. I humored them, thanked them for their concern, and never thought about what they said again.

Until I was in labor.

Nick and I agreed to explore labor in the tradition of Ina May Gaskin's *Spiritual Midwifery*. Gaskin says that a woman's labor can be stalled by anything from broken focus to bad mojo to unresolved latent desires. In this tradition, labor can be facilitated by a safe and inviting environment of the laboring woman's choosing, sexual/sensual contact with her partner, and a support system that emphasizes the birthing mother's needs.

The birthing mother, according to Gaskin, must allow herself to go there. As much as you might try to imagine where there is, it is unimaginable. Gaskin says that if all these things are in place, the laboring mother can have an ecstatic experience.

Along with the midwife, we had originally planned to have Gaby and our doula present, but I went into labor a week early and our closest friends happened to be staying over—Tony, Layla, and Steiner (the photographer)—so we invited them to join the labor party and document our process.

Nick and I did it all. We had the dimly lit room, we had a blow-up tub of warm water, we had music, we all walked in nature, we got naked, I shit in the woods, we nipple-stimmed, we did sensual stuff.

At first we did feel high—all of us remarked on it—like we had all taken Ecstasy (though I had never actually done any drugs besides weed).

Once active labor started, though, things got serious. Gaby and Nick remained by my side, while the others gathered by the hearth on the first floor.

During each contraction it felt like I was passing out and falling into this dense black space that both pulverized and pulled me apart. Inside it were pinpricks of white light with bone-quaking tremors—a literal earthquake in my pelvis—crushing the bones to powder, over and over again, for hours and hours and hours.

Nick and I fell briefly into a kind of hypotonic resting state, and in a pinhole of light at the end of the tunnel, I could see my midwife and her assistant—who was also her husband—slow dancing to the Grateful Dead; the husband was twice her size and had a long white beard and wore a fluorescent red and orange tie-dye shirt.

Both Nick and I thought to ourselves that we had made the greatest mistake of our lives.

The old retired gyno came for a visit in my head. "See?" he said. "You're going to die."

"Well, you were right, old retired gyno," I said back. "It was all hubris and the hippies steered me wrong."

After hanging off Gaby's shoulders while shitting and vomiting, I did a round of stair climbing at my midwife's insistence. Layla met me at the bottom of the stairs, and I wanted so badly to tell her about this black hole I was in, but no words came. I could barely see her.

Halfway back up the stairs I buried my face in my midwife's bosom and did it: I called out to my mother.

I was slightly self-conscious when I did it. *But this is the work,* I thought. This is the unresolved latent desire. Anything to get it over with, even calling out to Mom. *This is going there,* I thought.

Still, I didn't want literal "Viva" to show up.

I got back into the tub, and though the team was by my side, Nick in the water too, cradling me from behind, ultimately it was just me and the Singularity.

I dropped into the black hole and looked it in the eye.

The Singularity is the center of a black hole where extremely large amounts of matter are crushed into an infinitely small amount of space. In labor, this stage is called transition; it's when the cervix opens from seven to ten centimeters, and the baby begins her descent into the world.

Anyone who has given birth will tell you that you can, actually, exit from the other side of a black hole! And on the other side there is a tremendous ring of fire around silky wet hair on a little cone-shaped head that's ripping your pussy apart, and people are excited about it and they want you to look at it in a mirror and touch it. You want to say,

"You touch it, you fucking freaks," but you have no words because, you know, you were just dropped into a black hole and spit back out again, and all your atoms have been rearranged.

I don't tell my mother these details. I let her believe I was calling out to her physical presence to help lessen the blow of not being invited to the birth, but I still don't want her to see how much pleasure we took.

Still hovering dangerously close to the photo albums, she squeezes my shoulders. "You wanted your mommy after all, didn't you?"

"Yup," I say, trying not to shirk away.

After all, it was because of her that I chose to give birth like that. It was because of her that I had the confidence to insist on a home birth when everyone around us was warning us against it. So now I offer her an admission that she was wanted, that she was needed, that I had called to her for her strength and power.

Her phone rings. It's Fucking Marybeth, thank God. My mother forgets about the album as news comes in about the derelict nephews camping out on the land and building their own dock on the bay.

Meanwhile, I hide the album in the coat closet.

Chapter 11

As the World Turns

That baby coming soon?" Merle asked as I entered the lobby with some groceries from D'Agostino's. Merle was a resident who practically lived in the lobby because her actual apartment was a maze of stacked papers that reached the ceiling. She loved to chat with people coming through.

"My mother thought she was in labor, but then she realized they were Braxton Hicks," I said, hoping to impress the tourist sitting on the other side of the lobby.

"Just make sure you get her to the hospital in time," Jerry said from behind the desk.

"Labor takes much longer than everyone thinks," I said, hitting the gold elevator button.

Safely inside, I watched the numbers light up as it passed each floor, 5, 6, 7, pause, *ding!*, and I stepped onto the landing of our new floor.

Life was good.

"*Woo, woo!*" I called out.

The stairwell had a pleasant echo; I leaned over the banister and spit into the hollow vein of it. The globule floated down, past each floor, and landed with a dull splat on the cement slab where the stairwell ended, next to the black splats of gum and crunched wrappers. I took in the view of the center of the building, sweeping my eyes from the spit slab up to the huge, triangle-shaped, scummy glass sunroof above the tenth floor. Then I pushed through swinging doors with my hip and saw our bikes and some of our clothes strewn around our side of the hall.

Our new front door, number 710, was propped open.

My mother had successfully persuaded Stanley to give us a bigger apartment. It was perfect—a real apartment with a separate bedroom and its own kitchen and bathroom—high up enough for the "good light" to come through the windows in dusty rays, ghostly fingers reaching for us, trying to communicate something about the future—something I couldn't quite understand. Maybe they were warning signals cautioning me about the threats around us, threats that seemed to find my mother wherever she was—threats in the form of cabdrivers, strangers on the subway, deli counter men, joggers in Central Park who breathe too heavily too close behind her.

I stepped into our narrow entry hall and made a U-turn into the small kitchen—with black-and-white linoleum tiles just like the one from my video memories—where I put the groceries down and found my mother vomiting over the dishes I had just washed. I still found her very cute, though—she wore her hair in two short little braids, a purple velour jumpsuit and beige Wallabee shoes—but I did wonder: *Could she not have turned and vomited in the actual sink only a few inches away?*

Even when mildly irritated by her dramatics, I was still drawn to her pregnant body, compelled to rub and coddle her belly as though I were responsible for the baby's growth.

After she gargled with water, I crouched down and called up into her crotch—"Hey, this is your sister, Alex!"—in order to get the baby familiar with my voice.

My mother moved to the bedroom then, lying down on the bed and moaning. "Oh, God, Alex, you were so right about Patrick. How could I have fallen for such a pathetic excuse for a man? And Anthony. I can't even think about them."

The bedroom had the same view over the rooftops as the living room. The door to the bedroom had a frosted glass window stenciled with the word *emergency* in red block letters. My mother and I shared the hotel bed that came with the apartment; it had a metal frame that made my mother shriek "Goddamn it!" over the shin gashes and bruises it caused. Same with the bikes in the hall. Same with the sharp points of stucco paint on the walls, though the paint shredded our elbows more than our shins. My mother said she was going to make Stanley sand the walls down so they would stop destroying our arms, but while we waited for the sanding-that-never-came, we just nailed an old pilly and mustard-colored acrylic blanket to the wall behind the bed to protect the skin of the new baby once it was born.

My mother pulled herself up from the bed to go to the bathroom and vomit again.

Later that day she used her little black suction cup attached to the phone receiver to tape Anthony telling her that she was a manipulative cunt who got him stoned and seduced him into getting her pregnant. She played me the recordings afterward.

"Can you believe him?" she asked me while we listened together.

I was also thinking that actually the Wet Kisser might have been a better choice for a father than Fucking Anthony.

A few years back, when we used to hang out together at Barbara Steele's sunny white house in Hollywood, Anthony had seemed kind and friendly to us kids. I had assumed he was Barbara's boy-friend. Whenever they were alone together, Barbara and my mother would hoot about how cheap he was, so cheap he wouldn't even buy an extra bar of soap for his apartment. The cheapest man on earth, they said.

Now, apparently, he wanted nothing to do with us.

"Fuck him," I said.

Yet, still, we religiously watched *As the World Turns*. "Oh, what a total prick!" my mother would shout.

Lately James Stenbeck, Anthony's character, had been gaslight-ing Barbara, his TV wife, and we suspected that maybe he was get-ting his psycho character confused with his actual self.

"Oooh!" my mother howled. "They're really turning Anthony into a bastard."

The more of a bastard he was, the more vindicated we felt. We ridiculed their outfits and hairdos and all their furniture. We cre-ated a list of soap words and phrases—*you hurt me, I'm feeling vulnerable, I need some more time, I need you to be here*—and I would hold my mother's face in my hands, look into her eyes with mock drama, and say "You hurt me."

To PREPARE FOR the birth, I began studying the Frédérick Leboyer book *Birth Without Violence*. I examined the grainy pictures of women giving birth in water with the lights dimmed, their faces ecstatic, the gentle French doctor tenderly laying their newborns against their breasts with stiff dark nipples.

When I have my own child, I will have warm water, I planned,

I will have dim lights, I will have large swollen breasts. I strongly considered finding this Leboyer character and hiring him right then and there, just to make sure he would be secured for my future delivery. *You have to massage the perineum.* I took mental notes.

"Oh, these doctors rush everything, Alex," my mother said.

I watched her pull her black spandex low-cut Betsey Johnson dress over her belly. Her breasts bulged up from the low neckline, soft blue veins glowing under her translucent skin. This dress was my favorite—it pulled tight around her belly and then flared out over her small hips and slender legs. I fantasized about keeping the dress for my own pregnancy, but when I tried it on, it sagged across my chest and hips.

"They just want to get home as fast as they can, that's why they cut you. Honey, you can't imagine how corrupt these doctors are—especially the men. Well, all men are pigs. They can't help it. It's in their genes."

I wrote things down so I would remember what to buy and do when I was an adult: *I will have a girl baby with no father and my perineum will never tear. I will not be like the cranky pregnant ladies on the sitcoms; I will be like my mother: sexy and independent.* I made a list of what I'd need in one of my half-filled diaries:

velour shirts
Gloria Vanderbilt jeans
lavender eye shadow
a checkbook (must memorize how to fill out a check)
margarita on the rocks with salt
home birth in water

Her gynecologist, Niels, told her she couldn't have a home birth because she was forty-four. Because of her age, Niels wanted her to have an "amnio." Niels wrote a famous book for women called

Listen to Your Body, but my mother didn't trust him. She said he was a coke-head-mother-fucking sadist and probably a gigolo from the Riviera.

Despite her suspicions, she opted for the amnio. During the procedure, we gripped each other while they stuck a long needle right through her belly and into the uterus to get some of the fluid the baby was floating in. Afterward we rested, terrified. My mother had read that the procedure could incite a miscarriage, and so we prayed the baby would not dissolve and appear as blood, that the baby was healthy, but also, really, to find out if our prayers were answered and it was, as we suspected, a girl.

The call came.

"Uh-huh . . . OK . . ." she was nodding her head, expressionless.

I was about to explode with the suspense. "What?! What?!" I yelled out.

"The baby is fine," she whispered to me.

I almost fainted with relief.

"And the sex?" she asked the nurse. "Could you tell us what sex the baby is?"

I stared at my mother's face for her reaction. My palms were sweating. *Please, Fatima, please let it be a girl. If you love me at all, if you care about us, let it be a girl. I will do anything for you.*

And then my mother smiled. I knew what that meant. My body relaxed.

"Thank you," she said and looked at me, mouthing the words, "It's a girl."

WHILE WE WAITED for the baby to arrive, I began to venture out into the neighborhood by myself—picking up fruit and vegetables from the Korean deli across the street, serpentining to the Middle Deli to fetch late-night cravings (I feared random shootings from snipers, so I took the advice that Peter Falk gave to Alan Arkin in our new favorite movie—*The In-Laws*—and zigzagged while I ran so I'd be harder to target), and stopping by the Squat on my way home from school with Rebecca.

I soon found out that everyone at the Squat was part of a Hungarian theater troupe, a group of families who had taken over the entire building a few years before. They performed their plays in the theater space behind the storefront window, where a live goat sometimes slept on a paddock of hay inside. During performances, pedestrians would walk by this window and become, unintentionally, part of the show.

They had escaped communism, Rebecca explained to me, and her father was left behind to restore paintings in a big museum in Budapest. Or maybe he didn't want to join them, or maybe he wasn't invited. She worried she might never be able to go back to see him.

I was drawn to her story and also to the slightly awkward way she stood out from the rest of the kids. This was partially because of her height. We had height in common. I had never met a girl taller than me. It wasn't just that, though. She was an amazing artist, she had luxuriously wavy chestnut hair, bushy eyebrows, and dressed like she was from another time—brown velvet floral-printed capri pants with a zipper up the side. They seemed terribly old-fashioned and brilliantly avant-garde. I told her I loved them.

"Eva made them," she said.

I loved her mother. When I first met Eva, she excitedly jumped up and started clapping as though she had been expecting me. She made a whooping sound and wrapped her arms around me, giving me a fast, rough kiss on the cheek. She was captivating—tall and muscular with a buzz cut and a thick Hungarian accent. She fed me a fluffy spoonful of chestnut puree and scooted me down the hall as she called out: "Rebi! Here is Ahlex!"

But since my mother's belly was growing, I wouldn't stay away from home for very long—only allowing myself short visits to this strange and magical building before I returned to the Chelsea, to the pregnancy, to the baby, and to my mother.

EVERY TIME MY MOTHER LEFT the apartment, she would have to navigate her way through our narrow interior hall with her big belly, catching a piece of clothing on a handlebar, or scraping her shin against a bike pedal, or tripping over a random thing we couldn't find a place for in the rest of the apartment. This would send her into a frenzy of organization, which was really just her violently throwing everything into the outer hall and leaving it there for a while until someone complained, and then we would reorganize all of it and the apartment itself, going through the same rotation of living room setups—often using the big bookshelf as a dividing wall—because there were only so many configurations that could be had in one room with the same furniture.

During these reorganizations, her vent worries would always amp up.

The vent in question was on the wall in the apartment's hall, above the bikes, about three square feet, covered by an old wrought iron grating. The little openings between the curlicues of the iron were stuffed up with oily black dirt. Behind the grating was a cavernous black hole into which my mother often made Isaiah, the Chelsea's super (whom she really got along with), shine his flashlight.

She was convinced there was some kind of respiratory health hazard in there. I wasn't sure if Isaiah's flashlight would ever reveal the source of the hazard.

One Saturday afternoon I was lying on the living room floor studying the Leboyer book.

"I've been thinking," she said, looking up from the paper she was reading. "You've seen your own birth. You know how traumatic it was. I think we should take her home right after the birth. I can't let them put her in the nursery. That's probably why you had crossed eyes . . . Oh, I never should have let them take you away from me and put you in the nursery—I'm so sorry!"

I wondered what other kind of damage she suspected had been done to me.

"I won't let them stick her with needles and shove a bottle in her mouth with a thousand other screaming babies—it's barbaric. I was such a moron to let them do that to you. I'm coming home right after the baby is born. And I'll eat the placenta. It's loaded with nutrients."

Note to self: eat placenta.

"But we've got to get this vent cleaned out first," she said as she picked up the beige phone to call down to the desk and ask them to connect her to the basement. After a few beats she said, "Isaiah won't answer the phone. Honey? Can you head down there? I just can't take it right now."

I didn't love going down to the innards of the Chelsea where the superintendents had their own world. Over the last few months I had been down there a couple of times already to get Isaiah to help us with particular apartment issues, like when jiggling the toilet handle hadn't worked. But if I didn't go down myself, my mother could easily get into a lobby fight with Stanley about the vent and then he would get mad about the rent.

If I took the main elevators, I had to go through the lobby—where I might run into Stanley—and then through the lobby's phone room to get to the last flight of stairs to the basement. So instead, I chose the possible-plummeting-to-death route. Right across the hall from our front door was the door that led to a chugging, cavernous service elevator that felt as though it would yank itself off its cables and plummet through the basement floor at any moment. The garbage from each floor's communal bin traveled in this elevator, so its floor was permanently greasy and it stank of rotting broccoli.

That day I chugged down to the basement with Jerome, the bellman. He was in his loose brown suit. He offered me a tepid smile.

"Mom having that baby soon?" he asked.

"Any day," I said as the elevator clunked to a stop and spit me out into the basement, where the very low ceilings were draped with wires and pipes laced with cobwebs. Under pools of yellow light from the bare bulbs, men in jeans and tool belts sat at a large card table. They stared at me, stunned, like maybe I was an apparition.

"Is Isaiah around?" I asked, timidly.

"Here I am, little lady," he said, emerging from behind some pipes. I told him my mother needed him.

"No problem," he said. "Come on."

We got into the service elevator, and it started chugging its way back up to the seventh floor.

"Yeah," I said, trying to make conversation. "My mom's worried about the vent again. The vent, the vent, the vent!" I sang with a jazzy voice and did a little tap dance.

"Heh, heh. I'll take a look, little lady, don't worry."

It lurched to a stop, we exited, opened the back stairwell door, passed all our stuff piled in the hall again, and stood in front of our apartment. The door was propped open.

"Mom! Isaiah is here!" I called into the apartment.

"Oh, great!" she said, waddling out with her big belly.

She put her arm around Isaiah and directed him into our hall and pointed to the vent.

"In there," she said. "I'm worried about this filth. I'm sure we are breathing in black mold and toxins."

He pointed the flashlight into the vent but looked down at my mother's body.

"You look good, baby," he said to her.

I was surprised he was so into her pregnant body.

She smiled, coyly.

She had mentioned his tight jeans before, and I had thought they annoyed her, but now I could see they intrigued her. I wanted to tell them both that they reminded me of the mom and the super (Schneider) from one of my favorite shows, *One Day at a Time*, but my mother had said she couldn't stand Bonnie Franklin (maybe she was too much like the Unmarried Woman), so I didn't say anything.

When Isaiah left—no vent decisions were made—my mother called Ruth, our upstairs neighbor, to tell her about everything that had just happened in detail.

We could often hear Ruth yelling at her family through our bathroom pipes, which became her bathroom pipes, as our apartments had the same layout.

Whenever we heard Ruth's screaming through the pipes, my mother would roll her eyes and make the crazy signal with her finger at her temple and say, "Oh, God, there she goes again!"

I was tempted to say, *Just like you*, but instead I just rolled my eyes along with her.

Ruth had been an opera singer in Israel, so her voice carried well. She argued in Hebrew with her husband, Danny, and their son, Orya, who was a bit younger than me. Ruth was also pregnant, so she and my mother had a lot to discuss.

Ruth was a thumb-sucker, like me. That didn't stop me from judging her and promising myself that I'd never *ever* let myself suck my thumb as an adult woman, though. She sucked her thumb while she gave my mother advice about money, and sometimes, when we were particularly broke, she wrote us a check made out to "cash."

Over the years, Ruth and Danny had broken down the walls of the neighboring apartments—eventually adding on at least five more rooms to the original layout, gathering the little outer hall tributaries into their interior space until their apartment took over the entire back half of the eighth floor.

Ruth and my mother often called during their screaming fits to check on each other. If my mother was screaming, Ruth would call and say, "Vivalay, Vivalay," in her Israeli accent, "come upstairs. I make you some tea."

I loved it when my mother went upstairs. I would stay behind in our empty apartment for a bit, and relax, while keeping one ear trained on the ceiling and the pipes. I could hear them up there, pacing around and complaining, their voices rising with excitement and then bursting out into cackling laughter.

When the laughter started, I knew all was good and right and so I would head up to number 810, where Danny would be naked, like a hairy satyr, smoking a joint, and Orya would be somewhere in the maze of halls and rooms in the back.

I would hang out and listen to the women discuss things.

Ruth and my mother shared a belief in what they called scream-

ing. They thought it was healthy and good for the general community. My mother even wrote an article for *Vanity Fair* called "The
Woman's Scream."

I also loved it when my mom visited other apartments. She'd
leave a note for me on our front door with the apartment number
she was in. On the tenth floor I might find her having tea in the
wood-paneled library of the kind old composer and critic Virgil
Thomson, or hanging out in a room full of live reptiles with the
composer and conductor George Kleinsinger. Or I'd find her on the
third floor, lounging on the bed in a one-room apartment decorated
with empty Medaglia D'Oro coffee cans and curtains made of mul-
ticolored beads, laughing with Vali, a friendly Australian "witch"
and ex-muse of famous photographers, who had bright orange
hair and tattoos—black curlicues and dots—around her mouth and
eyes.

I especially loved hanging out at Shirley's apartment.

Shirley Clarke's apartment was entirely black and white—inspired
by Felix the Cat—and when I arrived, Viva would be sitting in a
chair by the desk under a poster from a movie that Shirley had
made, *The Cool World.* The poster had white words inside red circles: *Hooker! Fuzz! Junk! Rumble!* Shirley was across from her.
She was very small, had streaked black-and-white hair, wore smoke-
tinted glasses, and had a husky voice.

I would play with a stuffed Felix the Cat and listen while they
talked about men. My mother would say things like, "Oh, God, no,
Michel never touched me after I had Alex. No, he was always accus-
ing me of being middle-class. When I wanted to meet his family in
Paris, he was appalled. He would say, 'I had no idea you were like
zis.' He even rented his own apartment on the sixth floor so he
could fuck other women in peace! Ha!"

Shirley was on and off with a very famous jazz musician, and after a while one of them would say, "Poor Ornette," and I would perk up. I wanted to know what exactly they meant by this.

They adored Ornette Coleman, said he was a genius. A genius, my mother always said next, burdened with this . . . *thing.* As I put the puzzle pieces together I understood that maybe my mother had also had sex with him, or at least had *tried* to have sex with him, but couldn't because of the size of "it." Or maybe Shirley had just told her about it, I was unclear.

My mother had spoken before about the monstrous size of certain men's dicks; I had overheard her talking with her sisters about accidentally seeing her brother Johnny's "monstrosity." I didn't want to think about Johnny's thing, but I was intrigued by what other men had hidden in their pants.

"How big *is* it?" I once asked my mother about the jazz musician.

"Huge," my mother said. "Down to his knees. He once went to the emergency room and begged them to castrate him."

"What's that?"

"Cut if off."

"Oh my God! And so . . . what happened?"

"They circumcised him instead. But don't ever say anything to Shirley about this. Or him. We are not supposed to know."

When Shirley next brought up Ornette, I sat up straight and stared into the distance like I was hypnotized. "I like to watch," I said, deadpan. I wanted to change the subject in case I was tempted to say something.

My mother cracked up.

"Shirley, she's doing Peter Sellers!" she said.

"Oh, she's too much, Viva!" Shirley said.

I was imitating Chauncey Gardiner in the movie *Being There*, which my mother and I thought was the funniest movie we had ever seen. His character—a mentally disabled gardener who gets all his information from television but who everyone thinks is a genius—ends up staying in the White House or something, advising the president, spending time with a wealthy adviser's wife, played by Shirley MacLaine, who is trying to seduce him. When Chauncey says, "I like to watch," he means watch TV, but she thinks he is a voyeur, and so ensues a slapstick masturbation scene that had my mother and me laughing so hard, I fell off my theater seat.

As Christmas approached, my mother grew even bigger and more tired. When she moved in a certain way, I would ask if the baby was coming.

"Not yet, honey."

We hunkered down more often with the TV and called the bellman to fetch our nighttime cravings.

Calling the bellman was a delicate negotiation depending on who answered the phone at the front desk.

If Jerry answered, he often seemed annoyed, like we were not supposed to be using the bellman to do things like this.

Jerome kept things very simple—he was deadpan and kept his cards close to his heart.

Charles was more complicated and often drunk.

I tried to make it seem it was like all my mom's whims, and I had to follow her orders.

"Hi, Charles, could you go to the Middle Deli for my mom?"

"What you want? A Snickers?"

"Not a Snickers." I laughed. "But two pints of Häagen-Dazs?

One rum raisin, one strawberry? And those cookies . . . biscuits with the chocolate on top?"

Oh, God, I hated having to say their name: *"Petit Beurre?* You know, those ones my mom likes?"

"Petit Écolier," my mother corrected me in the background, overpronouncing the second word.

"Milk chocolate, huh? Naaah! Your mama wants the daaark, I know."

"Yes, please. Thank you sooo much!"

Eventually there was a knock on the front door, and one of us would answer it.

If my mother answered it, I feared she would say something like, "Oh, Charles, nooo! This is *milk* chocolate—look, read the package, right here, see?" like he was a kid. Then she might offer him a litany of complaints about things I knew he had nothing to do with. She might even send him back out for something! So I always tried to get there first, scrambling to get cash from the plastic egg (it once held nude pantyhose from Lamstons) that we kept in the top drawer. I prayed there would actually be cash in the egg because otherwise we would have to do a song and dance about paying tomorrow.

I didn't know where the cash in the egg came from, exactly. Some of it came in the mail as single dollar bills in sealed envelopes addressed to The Chelsea Hotel C/O Viva Superstar because when we were both on *The David Letterman Show* doing publicity for *The State of Things,* my mother asked everyone to send her a dollar because we were so broke, she said, because Andy Warhol never gave her a cent. David Letterman seemed angry and tried to end the show before she could finish yelling out, "Two-twenty-two West

Twenty-third Street! The Chelsea Hotel!" but apparently plenty of people heard.

One night, after we ate our Petit Écolier, I rested my head on her chest and stuck my thumb into my mouth.

One of our favorite shows, *Lifestyles of the Rich and Famous,* came on. We hooted and hollered over the bad nose jobs and tacky "homes." My mother hated it when Robin Leach said *home.* "It's *house!*" she yelled at the screen.

A lump pushed up into her belly skin. I pressed my fingertips against it. A tiny heel, maybe. It disappeared and then reappeared in a different location. I nudged it again and the lump moved across her belly like a cat under a sheet.

"I love thith baby," I said, my words garbled over my thumb.

"You don't know it yet," my mother teased, whacking my thumb from my mouth.

I stuck it right back in my mouth.

"Yeth I do," I said.

Chapter 12

Birth

My mother sat on the floor of our apartment moaning, breathing, and rocking herself through the contractions. She was wearing the purple velour jumpsuit, her hair in two braids.

This is it.

I was ready.

Once labor started, my mother had waited until the very last minute so she wouldn't be stuck at the hospital for too long. She went swimming at the Y and made a deposit at the bank. When she got home, she told me that the bank teller said, "Just don't have the baby in here, heh, heh, heh!"

I was supposed to be there, in the hospital room, for the birth, but Niels had decided I was too young.

"They're all fucking control freaks," my mother said. "I'm so sorry, honey, I should have *insisted* earlier that you *had* to be in the room."

Ruth and Danny helped my mother get to the hospital, and I stayed home alone to wait. They were supposed to check up on me later, but until then I had the apartment to myself.

Time stretched out over me like a heavy blanket. I tried to relax and focus on the fact that my dreams were unfolding.

Outside of the apartment windows, big fluffy snowflakes began to fall. I remained inside, waiting.

Somewhere out there my sister might have already left my mother's womb and entered the world. I would soon welcome her to our apartment, our world.

I waited.

We had studied the name book together.

"I think we should call her Fatima," my mother had said.

"No, Mom, that's way too obvious."

"Maybe Antonia?"

"Mom. Are you kidding? You want to name her after *Anthony*, the gaslighter? How about we just call her James Stenbeck?"

"Ha! You're right. I'm crazy!"

I liked boys' names for girls—like Frankie. My mother wanted more traditional names—like *Mary Antonia*. It was just like her to suddenly go nostalgic and old-fashioned and want to name the baby after her mother, who she said hated her, or Anthony, the psycho soap star.

We finally decided on Gabriella—Gaby for short. Gaby was my choice. It was a perfect name for who this baby would be, I thought. I felt like I knew her already. I had called the baby's name into my mother's crotch:

Gaby, Gaby, Gaby, I'm ready for you, baby, this is your sister, Alex. Can you hear me? It's me, Alex.

FINALLY, RUTH AND Danny came back and told me the baby had been delivered. They told me we were not allowed into the hospital, and the nurses didn't want my mother to leave yet, so we took a cab to Mount Sinai, stood below my mother's little hospital window on the third floor, and looked up. Big snowflakes landed in our eyes. My mother held the baby to the glass.

I tried to mentally span the distance and to tell them I loved them; I wanted to send my soul up through the window to bring them home.

I returned to the apartment again.

While I waited, I dropped a Barbie leg in the key shoot.

Finally, a knock at the door. I ran to it, clearing a free path through all the clutter. When I opened it, a clan of friends surrounded my mother, snow clinging to everyone's hats and coats, my sister somewhere in the middle. They moved to the bedroom like a school of minnows, and the baby was placed in the middle of the bed.

As I made my way through the bodies, the hospital bunting was unwrapped, and the clan parted, making room for me to see her for the first time. I leaned in close. I was finally face-to-face with her.

My heart sank.

She looked like Mel Brooks.

ONCE OUR FRIENDS LEFT and we were alone with her, our nerves crept in.

We began to worry the cold would kill her. So we closed the shutters and used our teeth to rip off strips of duct tape to seal out the drafts.

My mother lit a fire, and we turned out the lights and wrapped the baby in three layers. If we needed to unwrap her, we laid her down on a bed of pillows in front of the fire—quickly—blocking her from a runaway draft.

She was violet, squashed up, old looking, sort of limp, and pulsing like a skinned frog.

"Can you believe they didn't even clean the blood off me? The minute I told them I wanted to take her home right away, they just dropped me. That fucking Niels didn't even come back in to take the bloody pad out. They didn't want to be sued, I guess. I mean what do they think women do in the bush?"

"They're all crazy," I said, staring at the baby.

I was beginning to not mind that she looked not at all baby-like. Mel Brooks was actually my all-time favorite comedian besides Gilda Radner, Lucille Ball, and Carol Burnett.

"I'm still bleeding. I told them I wanted to squat, and that lazy bastard Niels wouldn't let me. I bet he didn't want to get his precious clothes dirty. Is it cold or hot in here?"

"I think it's just right."

My worries forced me to strengthen my reserve; I would not admit to being scared. But I was.

"Then they wanted me to sign paper after paper. I said 'Can anybody *please* give me a clean pad for the blood?' and they completely ignored me—can you be*lieve* it? Com*pletely* ignored me. Look—I've still got the hospital gown on!"

When the three of us got into bed, I watched the baby suction her lips onto my mother's tit and curl her toes. Her face was smoothing out.

We all got drowsy. I tried to keep my eyes open to watch her. When she stopped sucking, I pulled her into me. We fell into a light sleep, sweating.

I woke with a start: *Still breathing?!*

Yes.

My mother woke with a start: "Still breathing?"

Yes.

LATER, AS THE FIRELIGHT FLICKERED against the stucco wall, I woke when my mother tacked up another blanket to protect the baby from the sharp points of paint. I let my eyes close for a little while until I felt my mother moving again.

"I think it's too hot," she whispered.

She stood up on the windowsill and started peeling off strips of duct tape.

LATER STILL, I woke up. The baby was in the bassinet at the foot of the bed.

"I was afraid we would roll over on her," my mother whispered when she felt me leaning forward.

It must have been getting close to sunrise. I stared at the baby. She had become beautiful. Her face had turned creamy pink, and her tiny bow lips were translucent and plump.

"Crack a window too, honey. We need some air."

I climbed up onto the windowsill and pulled the shutters open.

Snow was still falling, light and slow, like white butterflies in the dark. The entire city was still except for pulsing blue televisions behind fogged-up windows. I imagined myself from outside our window, standing on the wide sill, hovering over the rooftops. I looked back at my mother and the baby sleeping—*the baby, my sister, Gaby, yes! That IS the right name, Gaby, Gaby, Gaby*—and my crumpled, empty space in the bed.

I love them! I wanted to yell out to my city. *Gaby! My sister!*

I breathed in deep, but I couldn't fill my lungs as much as I wanted to. I yearned to inhale the moment like druggy gas and encapsulate all the life contained inside the held breath, holding it forever. I filled my lungs with another deep breath, pasted a kind of frozen, camera-ready smile on my face, and whispered the sound: *chicka, chicka.* It was the sound of a camera shutter opening and closing, only I was the camera, or maybe the aperture.

Suddenly my mother sat up. "Darn it," she whispered. Her voice drew me back to the micro space of our bedroom. She rested her head back on the pillow and looked at me in the dark, still standing on the windowsill. "Those fucking nurses made me forget the placenta."

I crawled back into the bed and fell asleep with the baby's tiny mouth next to my ear. At sunrise I woke again and was awestruck by her breathy gasps that sounded like gentle *ah*s.

THE NEXT DAY friends came with flowers and Champagne. My mother looked calm and happy, thrilled to show off the baby.

Rebi and Eva were there. Eva insisted that we give her all the baby's dirty receiving blankets and onesies for her to wash by hand and deliver back folded in neat piles.

Rebi asked me if I wanted to come over. I hesitated. I looked at my mother and the baby surrounded by the audience. My mother was telling the birth story.

They will be OK without me for a short while, I told myself.

I whispered to my mother that I would be back soon, banking on her distraction, knowing she could barely digest this information.

I followed Rebi and Eva toward the door and looked back at my mother and the baby one last time.

Would they be OK?

The baby cried and my mother pulled out her breast.

The crying stopped.

Eva and Rebi were like Sirens; I felt a strange lethargy as I followed them out, like I was suddenly sick, but as we opened the lobby doors and exited into the icy January air, my blood quickened.

Leaving the shelter of the striped awning, we stepped into the brown slush, and Rebi and I began to run down the block, flanked by its four lanes of loud traffic, laughing, the cold biting our noses.

We didn't stop until we arrived at her building's storefront window, where I put my face to the glass and saw a fifteen-foot papier-mâché baby—with real TVs for eyes and a big plump vagina between its splayed legs—sitting in the dark theater, facing ascending rows of empty seats. Above the front door was a hand-painted sign that said Mr. Dead and Mrs. Free.

"I make hot chocolate," Eva said as she unlocked the door.

I followed them in.

Now

A light snow is falling. I push open our huge front door to watch Gaby approach the house. There she is—a whirl of frizzy chestnut hair with gorgeous gray streaks, and high cheekbones, like Viva's. Her eyes are deep brown with luxurious thick eyebrows like Anthony's. She wears no makeup, ever, on her alabaster skin. She's not as tall as me and not as slight as Viva. She's stunning, always.

Today she's elegantly wrapped in a woven cape-like thing, carrying her tow-headed, pink-cheeked cheery baby boy—Lewis—on her hip. Hanging off an arm are lots of half-filled cloth sacks with stuff spilling out—snacks, diapers, clothes, and a bottle of tequila. She never arrives empty-handed.

Closing up the car is her partner, Chris, another filmmaker. He is calmly tuned into the kids and just eccentric enough to remain patient and engaged with Viva during these family visits.

Viva is rarely cruel to Chris; they are still in the honeymoon period for reasons hard to pinpoint because he and Gaby have been together for more than a decade. Maybe it's simply because she admires Chris's youth and slim physique.

Nick is also a generous Viva buffer. After all these years of being maligned by her, he has somehow kept a reserve of love and enthusiasm for her funny side. Even for her crazy side—unless it really turns dark.

Rosy, Gaby and Chris's whip-smart, exacting four-year-old, is leading the way. When Rosy sees me, she jumps into my arms. While we embrace, I drink in her smell, and love her like my own.

Over Rosy's shoulder, Gaby and I exchange looks: *here we go.*

Miko and Lui seduce the kids away from me and take them into their own arms, and everyone moves inside.

Once inside, even a faint whisper about Viva can be dangerous. She has vigilant ears, almost magical in their ability to hear whispered words from far distances. Even our eyebrow movements could be intercepted and decoded.

"I know why you're looking at each other like that," she'll say. "You think I'm crazy."

When that happens, I employ the say-aloud-what-you-really-want-to-do-so-the-truth-then-seems-like-a-joke method: I grab my mother's shoulders, look her in the eye, and using a sinister voice, say: "Yeah, Gaby, let's lock her up in the loony bin and throw away the key, ha ha!"

When we are all together the dynamics shift, currents abruptly change. Without Gaby I was the morose, snappy "child." Now that Gaby is here, my mood has lightened; I'm freed from the compulsion to punish my mother, and I shift to being the merry prankster to make up for Gaby's taciturn mood and impatience with her.

Mom gives the kids their presents—dream catchers, geodes, and crystals. An Eileen Fisher–style cashmere wrap for Lui. They all adore the loot.

I make us margaritas. Gaby nurses Lewis.

Mom soon announces she is dying for chicken soup, and she is going to make some herself.

Gaby looks at me with wide eyes; I glance at Mom to make sure her back is turned, then I look up at the ceiling and pretend to be blinded by the sun.

Mom apparently looked at me while my eyes were squinted and busts me.

"What?" she says. "You don't want soup?"

"Oh no, no—the light was too bright," I say.

"The light? What light?" she asks, suspiciously.

This routine is meant to be done outside. Nick invented it. When Mom is saying or doing something funny/crazy/annoying—and you can't avoid reacting, but you don't want her to know you are reacting—you look up at the sun, squint your eyes, grimace dramatically, and say, "It's so bright!" But blaming the sun doesn't really work when you're inside.

Instead of answering her, I corral her into the kitchen while doing a vaudevillian soft-shoe dance and sing a Tin Pan Alley–style "Hello, my baby; hello, my honey; hello, my ragtime gaaaal! Yadda yadda yadda yadda yaaaadaaaa . . ."

Mom raises her eyebrows and flares her nostrils at me. She's not buying it. But she starts making the soup.

"We could order in tonight, Mom. My kids probably won't eat the soup," Gaby says from the living room.

Now that Gaby is a mother, her allegiances have shifted. She used to be preoccupied with taking care of Mom—she would have made the soup rather than let Mom tire herself out—but now she wisely tries to safeguard her patience and energy for her children.

"They'll eat the soup if I say so, right, kids?" Mom says to the kids with a mock dictator voice.

The kids run away screaming.

"Fako! Fako!" Mom calls after them with a fake whiny voice.

"Mom," Gaby says. "Can you not do that, please?"

When kids whine, Mom always says "Fako Fako." She did it to Gaby when she was a kid, and now she does it to our kids. It usually makes them whine more, but I've always been too chicken to ask Mom to stop doing it. Gaby is much braver than me.

Now that Gaby has asked Mom to stop, Mom is making a show of acting like she has to walk on eggshells.

"I'm just *kidding*," Mom says.

To be always just kidding—another absolution.

And then, in unison, we all finish her sentence for her: "Nobody gets my humor!"

While my mother starts the soup process, I unpack Gaby's bags. She inherited a bit of Mom's haphazard approach to packing and food storage. I pull out some onesies covered in loose oatmeal she bought from the bulk bins that have now spilled out of a torn bag. She's used to carrying a lot of stuff around. She's nomadic—at least in comparison to me. It seems Nick and I settle in one place for seven-year stints. Gaby is usually cultivating a few living spaces at the same time—a Brooklyn apartment, a trailer in the Catskills, a little house at the foothills of the San Gabriels.

I glance over at my mother cutting the onion: very abrupt, violent hacks, no pattern, chunks of onion landing on the floor. My skin tingles.

Soon comes the raw carcass flying around the kitchen, juice dripping over the clean dishes on the drying rack.

Ignore, ignore, ignore, I silently chant.

Then more of the violent grabbing and reaching. Chicken guts thrown onto a clean cutting board. The searching for pots with the gut-coated hands on the drawer pulls, the moaning about aging.

Nick is following behind her trying to wipe things down—which might agitate me more than the salmonella everywhere—while he says, "This is coo-coo-roo!" in a silly sort of ding-dong cartoon rooster voice he uses to diffuse tension.

Now the egg noodles must be had, and a trip to the store is sug-gested.

I try to distance myself from the soup, finding more complicated ways than Gaby had to suggest that making one of us go to the store for egg noodles means that making the soup is more work than it's worth and, at the end of the day, the soup is for her, not us.

I immediately feel bad about this and regret saying it.

She is proud of her cooking. Her soup would be the national dish if she were a nation. I used to believe it was the best chicken soup, but then very early on in our relationship, while eating the soup, Nick joked that my love of the soup was evidence of Stockholm syndrome, and the soup was actually a tasteless slop with shards of bones and branches of herbs and floating fatty globules. After he said that, I slurped some soup from the spoon and tried to be objective. It was bland and slick with fat. It had lost its magic.

Now I'm watching my mother jab the carcass into the pot like it's still alive and fighting back.

Chapter 13

Martyrs

For a while, we called her "the Baby." I was madly in love with her but exhausted.

I'd hold her in a patch of sun by the window, to relieve her jaundice, and pick the crud off her scalp, or the crust out of her eyelashes while she slept. I figured out how to distract her from nursing a bit longer by letting her suck on my thumb knuckle.

Her body—the weight of her, the smell of her—put some kind of spell over my mother and me so that just holding her made us not need or want to do anything else.

I was taking a bath with her when the scab from her umbilical cord fell off. Her belly turned smooth, round, and firm.

A shock of spiky black hair appeared on her head, soft like chicks' down.

In the dark parts of the early mornings, I insisted on taking the baby so my mother could get a little more sleep. Opening our apartment door and stepping into the hall was like entering the inside of a womb. A new soundscape. I would push through the swinging doors with my hip and leave our side of the hall, entering the stairwell hall, holding the baby. Under the fluorescent lights, I would jog up and down the marble stairs between the sixth and seventh floors. That kind of fast-paced jerky motion usually put the baby out.

Often, when I was doing the hall shift, a young couple would ding out of the elevators on another floor or pass me on the stairs as they returned to their room after a night out. They paid no attention to me—a kid jogging up and down the stairs with a newborn— I didn't hold their lack of interest against them—but I wanted them to know how precarious their carefree life was. I wanted to say, *You should appreciate these nights out, kids. One day you might have a baby to take care of, or my mother might come out at any moment and scream at you for making noise.*

When I heard the baby's breathing pattern shift and felt her body go heavy in my arms, I would check her reflection in the glass window of the swinging doors just to make sure her eyes were really closed. Often, when I stopped moving, she would stiffen and squirm and whimper, and then I would go jogging up the stairs again, my limbs burning with exhaustion.

I knew, though, that if I stuck with it long enough, I could get her in a deep enough sleep to sneak back inside the apartment, and ever so delicately lie down, keeping her close to my chest to secure a little more sleep for my mother before the next nursing session began.

WHEN THE BABY got a little more robust, I proudly took her to the deli in the fancy English pram my mother found (my mother was obsessed with English prams because she had one when I was a baby). The deli men nodded at me, respectful of my new status.

When I returned, a tourist held the lobby doors open for me, and I confidently popped the pram's front wheels up the step into the vestibule.

"Look at the proud new mother!" Jerry said as I crossed the lobby.

I watched the numbers light up above the closed gold doors as I waited for the elevator—4, 3, 2, 1—and that's exactly when I heard the whiny creak of Stanley's office doors opening.

"Uh . . . is that Alex?" he said, poking his narrow head around the corner to find me.

Fucker, I thought, cursing the slow elevator.

"I need to talk to you," he said, gesturing for me to follow him into his office.

With the baby?! I thought. *Jesus.*

I pulled the baby from the pram, left the pram by the elevators, and disappeared into the dusty room with piles of yellowed papers on every surface. The street-level windows were always covered by blinds. I sat in the big black leather chair at the corner of Stanley's desk, jiggled the baby, and gently dragged the toe of my shoe over the puke-yellow shag carpet, exposing the lighter underside of the yarn.

"How long have I known you, dear? Since you were born, that's how long. You're a sweet girl . . . You've really become a lovely girl. I don't know how you turned out so good with a mother like that."

I winced. If my mother had heard, she would have said: "As though I had absolutely nothing to do with it! Imagine! The imbecile!"

In the past, when we had these conversations, I would just humor him and tell him not to worry, that the money would come soon. But this time I felt my throat constricting and the pressure building around my temples, and I had to reach up and grab the bridge of my nose between my thumb and forefinger to stop from crying. Stanley didn't even notice. *Does he even see I'm holding a fucking newborn baby?!*

He continued, "But they won't have this. They will change the locks."

I had no idea who "they" were, but he was constantly talking about "them." My mother said "they" were bullshit.

"Look, Stanley," I said, "we have the money . . . it's just . . ."

"Alex? How old are you now?"

"Eleven. Same as last week," I mumbled and stood up, walking toward the door, hugging the baby close. I had the urge to swirl around, leap onto his desk and strangle him. "I've got to go . . . the oven . . . a . . . I have to go to the . . ." I said as I walked out.

"Well, if you don't talk to that mother of yours, *they* will, and she won't like it, I can tell you that much."

"OK, I'll tell her," I said, backing out the door. I never told her about these things. I didn't want her to go back down and start screaming at him about forcing a minor to listen to his bullshit.

MORE AND MORE I found my way to the Squat. I would soon start bringing Gaby along with me, but at first I used it to get some respite from new motherhood.

One day while I was waiting to be buzzed in, a woman in a tinfoil hat with a tinfoil penis on top stood at the inside of the storefront window, looking out. Outside, a crowd had gathered to watch when suddenly an army Jeep zoomed around the corner and screeched to a stop in front of the building; two men in fatigues jumped out, one had a disfigured face, and the other put his fist through one of the glass panes of the storefront; the crowd gasped; inside the theater's bright lights snapped on and the two crowds stared at each other—

the pedestrians and the official audience. After a beat everyone clapped and I was buzzed in.

I went right upstairs to Rebi's room, where we resumed our games.

We were *Little House on the Prairie* homesteaders surviving; we told each other stories; we birthed babies; we were dying women on the American prairie in the 1800s, saving our children from frost and famine. Or we were tattered women in some other century ravaged by war. The fact that it was actually freezing inside the building was great (the Squat often couldn't afford to pay the oil bill). We huddled under the loft beds, shivering, starving, trying to nurse our children as the bombs dropped. Sometimes we were going to a ball and one of us was a scullery maid, and the other was a bitchy rich girl. Galus, the daughter of the woman in the tinfoil penis hat, was always the prince we were fighting over. After the ball the three of us went up to the bedchamber (three tall loft beds in a row), where we dug ourselves under the heavy velvet quilts and "made love" to the men. For "the men" we used horsehair pillows that had traveled from Budapest. At that point we were each in our own separate worlds; I was finding the special place, the brief electric release from all worry and all dread.

Eva often made extra food—a goulash dinner or homemade gnocchi and chestnut puree—"For your moddair!" she would say, holding out a neatly packed paper bag.

Sometimes she would walk me home with a package made from a sheet tied tightly around the baby's hand-washed, ironed, and folded laundry. I was relieved we arrived bearing food and clean laundry because being gone for too long had been giving me an uneasy stomach. Had I been alone, I might have run up the seven flights, worried. Worried the baby would be fussing, or worse yet, that something bad was happening, like a lobby fight, or a phone fight, or something harder to pinpoint—a brewing mood.

Eva—so vivacious and breathy and hyper—made our apartment seem tiny. It was disconcerting to see her outside of the Squat, where she zipped around the big rooms, from floor to floor. Her neatly cropped hair, her hooded dark eyes, her wide face with creamy smooth skin and flushed cheeks seemed an extreme contrast to my mother, who was all wan and thin-wristed, frizzy-haired, blue-eyed, and pale, nursing Gaby under a painted portrait of Castro.

Eva hates communism, I thought. I was suddenly embarrassed about the portrait.

One night my mother said to Eva, "I don't know how you do it all," as she took the laundry from her.

Eva dismissed my mother's compliment with a cackle and skipped out the door.

"Eva is a saint," my mother said when the door closed.

She was eating the goulash. I was holding the baby, bouncing on the edge of the bed to quiet her.

"I don't know how she does it all," my mother said again. "Feeding all those junkies, making the sets, and taking care of all their kids. That's why your father took you there. To buy drugs."

I felt a twinge in my heart, but I kept a neutral face.

Junkies? I thought.

Eva was no junkie; that, I knew. The men might be doing drugs, I silently deduced, and it was plausible that my father was there to buy them. Rebecca had once suggested that there were nefarious interactions on the third floor, but I didn't ask her anything more about it.

It was my mother trying to slide bad things into my head that hurt the most.

THE SQUAT ASKED me to be in the revival of their play, *Andy Warhol's Last Love.* I would be Ulrike Meinhof—a Red Army militant and an assassin who shoots and murders the Warhol character at the end.

I was taking over the role from Eszter Balint, who was Rebi's stepsister of sorts (Eszter's father, Pisti, was Eva's partner). Eszter was a few years older than us, an intimidating teenager with an exotic brooding face. She looked like she was twelve but acted like she was fifty. She was famous in New York after having starred in a Jim Jarmusch film, *Stranger Than Paradise*, playing a character very much like herself.

Eva had made a lifelike rubber mask that fit over Pisti's head, and with the mask and the white wig he looked exactly like Warhol. My mother gasped when she first saw the costume and said, "Wow, Eva, that's pretty damn good." At times my mother seemed to admire Eva and the Squat, but then she could suddenly spin around and act like they were our enemies.

When they asked me to be in the play, I was terrified that my mother would say no. I was dying to do it, to be officially part of the troupe.

Eva called my mother to tell her about the rehearsal schedule, to coax her a bit, and promise that they would work around my ballet classes and my homework.

My mother agreed, but the more time I spent at the Squat—really any time I left the house—the mood I returned home to was off. My absence seemed to hollow something in her center, and literal hunger gnawed at her—she would always say: "I'm just starving!"

To make up for my absence, I began to bring Gaby along with me as much as I could. At the Squat she could play with Cora, one of the little kids from the third floor. This, I felt, would balance the scales, though I was beginning to wonder why we had a scale to balance in the first place.

Sleepovers were the hardest things to get away with.

One day I returned home from spending the night at the Squat, and I found my mother in a frenzy, pulling everything out of the closets. This didn't bode well for the slumber party I was supposed to go to the very next day, so I had to figure something out.

I settled on telling her I was really excited about taking Gaby to her first slumber party and that the friend's mother had already agreed. Luckily, my mother didn't question this.

When I arrived at my friend's door with Gaby in the Snugli baby carrier, her mother looked shocked. She said, "Oh. Will the baby be sleeping over too?"

"Oh yeah, she loves it. I do this all the time."

I managed to navigate most of the party with the baby. Once all the kids were sleeping, though, Gaby began to reach into my shirt to nurse. She had done this before, but usually my mother was nearby to give her the real thing.

I tried to distract her by tickling her back. I snuck into the kitchen to get her some milk. But once she started to cry, she wouldn't stop. My friends began to wake up. I felt frantic, though I pretended not to be worried.

My friend's mom woke up. She seemed genuinely concerned. I was embarrassed. She hailed Gaby and me a cab and handed the driver some cash.

"I guess she's not ready for a sleepover yet," my mother said when she greeted us at the door and took Gaby from my arms to nurse her.

I wanted to cry—from exhaustion and disappointment—but I just said, with a cheery voice, that maybe next time it would be easier.

I had to be very careful about complaining. If I did complain, she would fixate on the thing I was upset about. If I had said that the other mother seemed annoyed I brought the baby, or that I was upset about the whole thing, she might call that mother and yell at her for "kicking us out" in the middle of the night.

Same for the play. I tried to make sure to never complain aloud of being tired after a rehearsal. I slipped up, once, and said I was too tired to finish my homework. My mother immediately said she wasn't going to let me do the play anymore.

"They're using you, those Hungarians," she said.

"Please, I beg you. I want to do the play. I'm actually not tired at all, I was just saying that. I can't just drop out . . ."

"I'm telling them if you don't get home by ten, that's it. I'm not kidding."

"But, Mom, the rehearsal doesn't start until nine thirty! They need me to be there!"

"Too bad. Why doesn't Eva that fucking *martyr* stand in for you, huh?"

I wanted to scream at her: *Martyr?! Look who's talking?!* But I didn't. I had to manage her correctly. As long as I took Gaby with me, as long as I helped as much as possible around the house and stuck to the rule—never complain—she couldn't stand in my way.

Chapter 14

Press

When I took Gaby out for walks and errands in the Snugli, I soaked up the admiration from strangers. I liked how capable I looked. "Is she yours?" people asked. Depending on my mood, I said either one of these two things: "Yes, she's only three months old. I'm a single mother" or "Ha ha, yeah, right—I'm only twelve."

As the first two years of Gaby's life unfolded, I admired my mother's mothering of a baby, and then a toddler. She was not a planner. She was not a scheduler. We ridiculed those who were. We ridiculed Dr. Spock and all the baby books and all the mothers who worried about schedules and sleeping and when to feed the babies food and all the mothers who had baby rooms and cribs and monitors. Our baby nursed whenever she wanted, slept in our bed, and lived a schedule-free life. We rolled our eyes when other mothers at the playground complained about how early their children woke up. We thought: *Well, don't put them to bed so early, duh*. If Gaby wanted to stay up until midnight singing into her plastic mic—we let her!

But when my mother was angry, I wanted to collapse on the ground and sleep forever. Once we were on our way to a lovely day in Central Park, where my mother would paint the cherry blossoms and Gaby and I would wrestle in the grass. As we crossed the street, she reached both arms out like she was either casting a spell or conducting traffic. A left-turning truck driver didn't obey. Her knees buckled with rage, and she crouched in the middle of the crosswalk and screamed, "Mothers and children have the right of way you fucking cocksucker!"

Even if I had a paddock of hay to collapse on, I would never let anyone know I was mortified. I was stalwart. I stuck by her and tried to make sure the truck driver didn't kill her when he stepped out of the cab with his fists cocked.

GABY'S BLACK HAIR FELL OUT, and fluffy honey-colored ringlets came in. A psychic told my mother that Gaby was the reincarnation of Shirley Temple, and my mother believed her. I was suspicious of the psychic, though I did think Gaby was really smart and I had to admit she sometimes acted like Charlie Chaplin in the crazy dictator movie.

I recorded Gaby's firsts in a homemade book I bound together with yarn. I numbered her first words and neatly printed them in ink:

1. Hot
2. Penis
3. Bitch
4. I love you
5. Fuck

6. Wompah Woom (*Romper Room*)
7. Fouwah (four)
8. Cwazy (Crazy)
9. God
10. Fwaggle Wock (*Fraggle Rock*)
11. Balls (the toys, not the human anatomy)

We had a family portrait taken around the television set. My mother and I stood behind the television, I held Gaby, and my mother directed the photographer to wait for one of Anthony's close-ups before the shutter clicked.

Newsweek printed that and another picture of the three of us on the Chelsea roof, looking triumphant. Underneath the picture was an article talking about how the actor Anthony Herrera wanted nothing to do with his daughter. We read it aloud to each other proudly, and then my mother cut out the article and put it in her Publicity file under the name: Anthony's Refusal to Acknowledge Paternity.

IN ONE OF OUR ATTEMPTS to make the apartment feel more spacious and novel, I briefly created my own bedroom in the storage space above the kitchen, accessible by an old wooden ladder. When I was sitting up, my head barely cleared the ceiling. It had enough room for a single foam mattress and a Barbie house. It was short-lived because I soon discovered that when my mother cooked dinner, it became a human-size pizza oven. Still, I was excited to have my own private space. I drew all over the walls and wrote *"Micheal" J. Fox* with a heart next to his name.

One night after Ken and Barbie got naked and humped, my

girlfriend and I wedged ourselves into the coffin-like sleeping space and re-created the scene. As I rubbed my pelvis against hers, I heard a creak below. I quickly rolled off her, crawled to the foot side of the mattress, and peered over the edge. From above, I watched my mother's frizzy hair floating from the fridge to the sink and then out of the room again.

I crawled back on top of my girlfriend, hoping the mood hadn't changed, and began again. The rush of excitement was blinding; I held my breath so as not to pant in her face, but just before the relief came, she said: "*Stop.*"

"Yeah, we better go to sleep, ha ha," I said.

I quickly rolled off her, ashamed by my eagerness, and by the beads of sweat rolling off my forehead—though the sweat may have been from the heat of the oven below.

Soon after, when I moved out of the storage space, my mother bought bunk beds and gave Gaby and me the bedroom and moved her bed into the living room.

We could hear her on the phone, as usual.

"I know, I know, I mean it's all so disgusting, so ludicrous. Anthony makes thousands a week on that soap, and we get one hundred and seventy-five paltry fucking dollars. They all knew him too. At family court. They waited on line to get his autograph. Even the clerk. Thousands! *Oh, they make me sick those bastards at family court.* They all watch him on the soap. Even those cunts at social services are out to get women. We waited on line for two hours . . . hold on a minute," she said as she opened the emergency door to check on us.

I kept my eyes closed and my breath steady so she would think I was asleep.

"Good, they're sleeping," she continued. "Dita, you wouldn't be*lieve* the scene there—a bunch of fucking cunts. Finally, I just sat down and sobbed and begged for a glass of water, and one woman took pity on me. I'm serving Anthony with papers."

But this bedroom setup didn't last long either. With her bed in the living room, the sounds from the hall kept my mother awake at night. Couples or groups of people would be returning from a party, or a club, or who knows what, and they would be lollygagging in the hall, their laughter and gossip and howling bouncing off the marble and into our apartment. My mother took it like a blatant insult. I thought about going out into the hall in my nightgown and pleading with them to quiet down just to spare us all—especially themselves—the ensuing scene. I wanted to say: *You have no idea what you are getting yourselves into by continuing to enjoy yourselves in this public hallway.*

Sometimes she would bang on the apartment door from the inside and tell them to please let her children sleep. Then, if they didn't quiet down immediately, she would bang on the door again and yell, *"Shut the fuck up!"* with a shrillness that always surprised me because the moment before she screamed she had sounded completely normal. It was like the act of banging on the door had driven her mad.

If they still didn't quiet down, she might actually try to storm into the hall. To thwart her, I made sure to use the steel rod. It was some old-fashioned thing the Chelsea doors had—a thick rod that fit into a notch in the floor and another notch on the door. Having to unlatch the rod would slow her down significantly.

Other times she'd scream, "I'm calling the police, you assholes!"

About half an hour later we would hear the hollow scratchy voices of the walkie-talkies echoing in the hall, and I'd unhook the steel rod and open the door for them, still nervous, because I didn't trust that the police could control her.

"Oh, it's always something in this fucking hotel, officer. This whole place is riddled with drug dealers, whores, and gigolos keeping me up all night. Officer, I'm a single mother of two. I'm breast-feeding. I can't take it anymore!"

When she said, "I can't take it anymore," her voice would suddenly go quivery and shrill, and she would burst into tears. Her body would shake from the sobs and the sobs would quake, uninhibited, out of her body.

While my mother's outbursts weakened me—my limbs went both hollow and heavy—Gaby's two-going-on-three sense of self emerged full-bodied and forceful. She was like a little wood troll performing a spell on Mom, standing below her, demanding, "Stop it, Mom! It's OK . . . don't get cwazy! Gawd!"

Because of the hall noise, we moved Mom's bed *back* into the bedroom, wedging it between a wall and the foot of the new bunk beds.

To get down from my top bunk, I had to hook a heel in one of the ladder notches and jump onto her mattress below.

To get up, I had to step on the foot of her bed, hook my toes into an upper ladder notch, and catapult myself up to the narrow mattress.

From up there I could see my mother's frizzy hair when she was lying in bed, and I could hear Gaby's breath below me.

BECAUSE WE WERE used to the sounds of police walkie-talkies in the hall, on the night of the big fire we didn't wake up until the firemen were pounding on our door. I was the first to realize something more serious was happening.

I jumped off the top bunk onto the foot of my mother's bed, onto the floor, and ran to open the front door, where I struggled with the steel rod.

I screamed out for my mother and Gaby to wake up.

When I finally got the door open, smoke poured into the apartment from the hall.

"Out this way!" I heard someone yell through the smoke. One of the firemen grabbed my arm and pushed me forward; my mother trailed behind, holding Gaby, all of us in our nightgowns.

The fireman escorted us down the central stairwell. The smoke was so dense that it was hard to see the stairs. He held my hand and I held my mother's hand. Water dripped on my head from the tenth floor skylight, which had been smashed open to let air flow through the building.

"I can't breathe, I can't breathe," I said, pulling on the fireman's arm. He put his mask over my nose. Then he pushed us toward the last landing, where the water had flooded the hall. As we waded through the water, a fireman stumbled into the hall, ripped open his jacket, and fell into the water, vomiting.

In the lobby lots of people were gathered, smoking cigarettes, gossiping.

The glass doors were propped open, sucking in cold air.

Gaby didn't seem bothered at all; she was laughing and talking to our neighbor Merle.

"Put this on, sweetie," the lady whom my mother suspected was a call girl said, handing me one of her fur coats. There was glass shattered on the lobby rug, and the huge print of a woman with a tear falling out of her eye had fallen from the wall.

Gaby opened the lid of the red coffin and crawled inside, as I had taught her to do.

Stanley was giving the police a "statement."

My mother paced behind him.

Her movements were making me tense. She had this arch to her lower back and a shapely ass—which she was proud of—and she let it jiggle when she was relaxed, but she was stiff and her wide-set blue eyes pierced into the back of his head.

"This is disgusting," she was saying, "this is insane! We can't live here anymore, we *just can't* live here. I'm not paying the rent this month. Did you hear that, you slumlord?"

I pulled the sleeve of her nightgown and said, "Mom, it's OK."

We were finally allowed back into our apartment.

In the morning the *Post* headline, January 16, 1984, said: "Actress and Kids Flee Fire: Viva's 13-year-old daughter, Alexandra, says 'Everything is fine.'"

The three of us were there on the cover, sitting on the vinyl bench, looking forlorn. Inside there was an article about my mother and a picture of her from her movie *Lonesome Cowboys*. I stared at the picture. She was made-up, frizzy-haired, and sexy looking.

I read the article a few times over. It said something about how Viva was a "high-cheek-boned Botticelli beauty" and how she was once described as a "hippie Dietrich and an outgoing Garbo."

My mother nonchalantly clipped the article and slipped it into a folder labeled Press, next to some other folders with labels like Couches and Genital Mutilation.

We were filed away now, the three of us together, suspended in that moment in the lobby. I was excited to be in there with her. In there with her other selves who were filed away—a clipping of her on the cover of *The New York Times Magazine* with Andy Warhol and a clipping of a Diane Arbus portrait in *New York* magazine that she loathed because she said Diane intentionally made her look like a hideous drug addict. All the selves filed away gave me a pleasing feeling of delineation and order. I could just open the metal drawer and examine my mother at a particular moment in a particular time.

But it was hard to reconcile the paper-thin clippings with the living, breathing being standing in front of me. I was proud of her fame in the filing cabinet, but what did the woman in the drawer have to do with my mother?

That week a man stopped us in front of the Chelsea and said, "Are you Viva Superstar? I just saw you in the paper. I idolized you in the sixties! I even named my dog after you! I thought everyone from those days had OD'd. I'm so glad you and your girls are OK!"

My mother was a close talker. She leaned in when she said, "Oh, I never did drugs; that's all a myth. It's funny how everyone thinks we were on drugs—nobody was high in the movies I made."

The man said "Wow" and walked off with his dog, Viva.

"What an asshole," she said as we entered the lobby.

Now

She is attacking a long sheath of white drawing paper.

"I'm going to paint with the kids. Where are those brushes I sent you?"

I tense up. Dread creeps in.

Let her do her thing, I coach myself. This is her forte. Art with the kids! Stay out of it.

She is aggressively prodding the art supplies.

"You probably threw the brushes out," she says, matter-of-factly when I don't reply.

"Oh my God, of course we didn't," I say.

But where are those fucking brushes?

If she had sent us a fifty-cent dream catcher forty years ago, she would want us to be able to locate it immediately. Once she sends us something, she starts calling us about it, telling us when it should arrive, asking if it has arrived yet. Everything that arrives is protected from inclement weather and thieves by a box sealed in a pound of packing tape and notes written all over it in her big loopy cursive: *DROP AT DOOR. FRAGILE. FOR MIKO. DO NOT LET PAINT DRY ON BRISTLES. LEAVE BOX IF NO ONE ANSWERS.* She also loves to have things sent *to* her. After a visit, I'll get a call about something she left behind, something she needs me to find and send back to her, something like a single disintegrating water shoe. "Did you find it, honey?" she will ask. "No, it's not here," I will say, looking right at it, because, unlike her, I'm allergic to the post office.

Now she starts frantically pulling stuff out of the art cupboard and throwing it to the floor.

I'm proud of the art supply cupboard, though the kids rarely use it.

"Here they are!" she yells. "And they're ruined!"

She is holding out the brushes she sent months ago—now caked with dried-up red acrylic paint—like severed heads.

"Miko, you have to clean the brushes right after you paint, or keep the bristles in water!"

I look at Miko and smile. I say with my eyes, *Don't worry about it, nothing is ruined*, though if my mother weren't here, I'd be haranguing him about the same thing.

She arranges Rosy and Miko with the white paper and selection of acrylic colors on a plate, and she draws them while they paint. She's wearing a down coat and a hat with ear flaps.

I realize I'm nervous because she might start arguing with the kids. *Let her do her thing with the kids*, I remind myself again. She's great with kids, right? When I had Lui, I still believed she was magic with babies.

When Lui was a newborn, she had colic—or whatever it is we now call the inconsolable crying of babies. I was also inconsolable when nursing her didn't work. I thought I knew everything about raising an infant. If you give the babies what they want, my mother had said, when they want it, they'll be happy. Wasn't that what we said when Gaby was born? But that "method" wasn't working!

My mother arrived to help. She seemed worried about Lui's cries. I thought she would be mellow, unperturbed by any of these postnatal hiccups.

"Maybe you are eating too much garlic; don't eat anything spicy;

maybe she's allergic to your milk; maybe she's in pain; maybe we should take her to the doctor. I'm worried," she said.

I didn't want her to worry. Her worrying was making things worse.

I was worried too, but I wouldn't admit it. I dismissed everything she suggested while secretly being terrified to eat garlic.

I had imagined I would be the capable new mother showing everyone how it's really done—teaching yoga while wearing the baby in a sartorially successful wrap *while* the baby nursed and I engaged with the world without ever even mentioning the demands of motherhood.

I was not at all this version of a new mother.

"You never cried," my mother finally said after Lui sobbed for some time.

I never cried? Well, then, what is this right here at the back of your book where it says that in order to get me to stop crying, Michel—excuse me, I mean Frederick—rocked me to sleep in a taxi?

"Gaby never cried either," she added.

Oh, really? So why was I jogging up and down the Chelsea stairs with her at three a.m.?

Once the colic ended, Lui was easy. When she was a toddler, we lived on the same block as my mother in Venice, California. The way she let Lui dictate the flow could be magical. Lui wanted to take forty-five minutes to climb three steps? No problem! I felt genuine tenderness for my mother when I saw her harvesting loquats with Lui in her backyard and letting Lui guide her through the neighborhood—Lui's little pointer finger leading the way—while she followed behind, pulling the red wagon she had filled with Lui's stuffed animals. Then again, we might return home from the movies to find her pulling Lui around Venice in the wagon at one a.m. Reason being? Lui insisted.

Let them do what they want, and they'll be happy.

"Aren't you hot?" I now ask her as she paints Rosy and Miko.

"Shh! You don't know what it's like to be old," she lowers her voice and gestures to Miko's painting, a whirlpool of red. "He's on a roll—we have to take it away at just the right time, before he ruins it."

"I know when I'm done, Fafa," Rosy says, refusing to accept Grandma's curatorial intervention.

"Ooooo!" my mother shoots back, sounding like she just touched something very hot.

Rosy gives her a disapproving look.

Chapter 15

I Spit on Your Grave

Rebi and I were inseparable. We were at the same Junior High School—IS 70—just a few blocks away on Seventeenth Street. We walked home together every day, past the guard at our dreary public school, past a tuft of hair blowing along the sidewalk like tumbleweed—evidence of another girl-gang fight—past the magazine/candy/cigarette stand where we would buy a single cigarette for a dime and smoke it on the corner. Rebi was almost six feet, and I was just a couple of inches below. I, too, was now wearing velvet pants that Eva had made for me. We were not popular, but we didn't care; we did our own thing, had our own shit to deal with.

One afternoon, after I left Rebi at the Squat, I entered the apartment to find my mother holding the phone to her mouth, not to her ear—never a good sign. Her voice was spilling out, ice cold.

"Michel," she was saying into the phone, "your daughter wants to tell you something." She held it out to me, shook it. "Tell him. Tell him what you saw. Tell him! Tell him he's a junkie and you know it."

My throat filled with cement. She stared at me and waited.

There was an immutable silence between us as we stood in the living room, her eyes boring into my head, mine staring at the floor. After what seemed like an eternity, she brought the receiver slowly back to her mouth.

"What she won't tell you," she hissed, "is that she saw your drugs."

She held the phone out again to me and shook it again. It was hard to distinguish my father from the plastic receiver.

"Tell him, Alex. I mean it. *Tell him*."

I stared at the receiver, then at her, then at the receiver again. The cement had traveled from my throat down through the interior of my body, arriving at my feet and dragging me down to the bottom of the ocean. The outer shell of me was still there standing in the living room like a cardboard cutout.

"It's all my fault, right?" She was talking to both of us, the phone still outstretched between us, her voice loud enough to be heard in the outer hallway. "Everything is my fault, everyone blames the mother. Tell him!" She turned shrill. "Tell him!"

From the bottom of the ocean I could still send signals up to the cardboard cutout. I accepted the phone, untangling the beige cord in order to get the receiver to my ear.

"Dad?" My voice was weak.

"Listen." He laughed nervously. "Zat's nossing—zat's nossing, Alex. Your mozer is crazy. It is codeine for my toose . . . What did you see?" he finally asked. The signals were weak, making it hard to pull the words out. "I know it's nothing," I said. "I know—"

My mother yanked the phone away fast and hard enough to scuff my ear.

"You fucking *bastard* . . . ," she seethed into the phone, and then he hung up on her.

She continued to scream for an hour or so while I'd retreated to the bedroom.

Gaby stayed with me there, periodically opening her huge brown eyes wide while she lifted a thick eyebrow in a curious way, like she was expecting something funny to happen. I held her hand and rolled my eyes, trying to make light of it so she wouldn't think I was too upset.

Mom came through the bedroom on her rounds, shoving clothes in drawers, ordering me to get the dirty laundry together, saying that she was sick of living in the pigsty-postage-stamp apartment. Most of all she was angry that I was constantly running to my father's, that kids never call their fathers to task, that no one ever thinks it's the father's fault, that I am never home, that she can't do everything.

I'd love to know what you would do if I actually wasn't ever here, I thought to myself.

I had begun to talk back in my head more and more.

I WOULDN'T HAVE ADMITTED IT aloud, but it was true that I was "constantly running" to Michel's, although now it was Michel and Cindy's. Cindy was his new girlfriend. I'd met her the weekend he told me we would be sleeping at her place—a walk-up loft on Fulton Street where the toilet was in the communal hall and the shower was in the kitchen. When she answered the door, I knew by the way she smiled at me that she wanted to love me.

She was shorter than I was, soft-spoken and giggly. She had small features and tender blue eyes.

I loved her back.

She was an artist, my father had said, and I was moved when she showed me that she had turned her studio area—separated from the living space by a curtain—into my temporary bedroom. There I had a blow-up mattress in front of a large photography backdrop surrounded by professional lights from a movie set and disguises hanging from the wall organized by category.

Cindy was compulsively organized. She had neatly lined up rubber noses—some warty, some hooked; pig snouts and plastic boobs—small and pointy, huge and drooping; wigs in every color and style imaginable; latex asses—some pimpled, some wrinkly. File drawers were neatly stacked with googly eyes, fake eyelashes, fake teeth, and enough makeup to open a store. A rack of costume dresses formed one of my bedroom walls.

She would spend hours transforming herself into characters—gluing on the noses, choosing the right wig, smoothing the plastic boobs to her chest so the seam was almost invisible, and applying makeup in a way that made her actual face unrecognizable. Once she had turned into one of her characters, she would take pictures of herself by discreetly stepping on a button fastened to a rubber tube attached to her camera.

Cindy introduced me to her love of horror movies like *Night of the Living Dead, The Texas Chainsaw Massacre,* and *I Spit on Your Grave.* Even though she was obsessed with horror, she cried at the drop of a pin and was devoted to a blind dove with crusted eyes named Birdie, whom she kept in a little open box next to her bed. She had a hard-core irreverence, a sweet voice, and a tenderness that soothed my heart.

I started bringing Rebi along with me, eager to share the novel experience. Cindy welcomed Rebi and encouraged us to dig in to her treasures. We dressed ourselves up like white-gloved ladies from the 50s and she took pictures of our scenarios. We were inspired by her work and re-created some of the characters from her series of photographs she called Untitled Film Stills.

On Saturday nights the three of us would cozy up on her little couch and eat pints of ice cream while we watched people with sewn-up leather-skin faces chasing teenagers, limbs spurting blood, and ravaged women zombies walking in the woods. My father would be across from us in the kitchen area, making food, diddling around, filming us.

They seemed happy.

I suspected he still crinkled his paraphernalia, but I couldn't tell if Cindy knew or even if I was imagining the whole thing altogether. I was unclear about their arrangement, but I preferred to not dig in because I looked forward to these weekend vacations where Cindy created an escape that asked nothing from me.

I didn't want to disrupt it in any way.

MY MOTHER WAS AGAIN STANDING in the living room holding the phone out toward me when I got home from school.

"Here," she said as I put down my book bag, dreading what was coming next. "Your *father* just got married and didn't even invite you."

I exited my body and took the phone from her.

"Nobody came to dis wedding," he explained. "It is just signing some papers. At ze city halls."

"I know, I know," I said, trying to inject life into my voice. I felt the thud of betrayal in my chest, but I forced myself to smile, averting my eyes from my mother's scrutiny, playing it off like it was my mother's drama that I had nothing to do with. That made her grab the phone away from me and yell some things at him.

"Typical, she's thirty," she said when she slammed the receiver down. "Not even telling his own daughter first. *His own daughter!*"

"I don't care, Mom, *God!*"

"Well, you should care. Does Cindy know he's a junkie? I think you should call and ask her . . ."

It was a good question, actually, one that I wouldn't ask, but, again, I would never *ever* admit this to my mother, and I still much preferred willful ignorance in exchange for luxurious weekends with Rebi and Gaby at the country house that Cindy rented upstate.

In return for their unquestioning open arms, I didn't even wonder why they hadn't told me ahead of time, why they hadn't invited me to city hall. It was possible they were protecting me from my mother's reaction, or protecting themselves, but it was also possible they hadn't even thought to tell me beforehand.

After my father and Cindy got married, they soon moved into a much bigger loft in Tribeca, with one room for the toilet and another for the bathtub and shower. They built me my own room above the kitchen with a real set of stairs and a desk. The back of the loft was both their bedroom and Cindy's huge studio—all her disguises stored in custom-made cupboards. There was also a trapeze and a Ping-Pong table.

From my loft above the kitchen I was soothed by the sounds of Michel and Cindy collaborating on dinner together, laughing, and calling each other poopsie. I would willingly come down to help with dinner before they ever asked me—smash garlic cloves and make Michel's salad dressing the way he had taught me. After dinner I always offered to do the dishes, but they told me to leave it to them if I had a lot of homework, or they would insist I relax when I was tired after ballet.

When I was there, my mother started leaving ranting voice

messages on the answering machine. When Cindy pressed PLAY and my mother's voice suddenly cut through the loft and seized my soul, Cindy would immediately stop the message. I was grateful for this.

Once, after Cindy was unable to turn the volume down fast enough, my father snapped, "What is your mozer, drunk?!"

My defenses sprang, stinging my eyes, but I didn't respond. I wanted to say: *Of course she's not drunk. Do you really think she is that kind of mother? That she gets drunk and yells? She just yells because she . . . she has to . . . she's overworked, she needs money, she's . . . she's not drunk!"*

"Ignore it, she's crazy!!" he yelled at the machine.

Cindy rubbed his back and said, "Don't worry, poopsie, it's OK."

I was amazed at how calm she was. I had never seen anyone react to anger with kindness.

My father then slipped behind a partition off to the side of the living room where he kept his video equipment.

From my bedroom I could see a sliver of his back when he was sitting at his desk. Each time I heard a crinkling or a snort, my senses sharpened.

Was he still doing it?

Everything I observed told me yes, yet they both acted completely normal, so I questioned my own suspicions. But then he would be gone at odd hours, and he would still swipe his nostrils with his fingertip and run the same fingertip under his upper lip.

Maybe it was a tic he couldn't get rid of? Cindy would never be OK with a drug addict, would she?

I couldn't answer these questions, so I sealed my insecurities and confusions away; first, so my mother couldn't get to them; then, from myself.

"WELL, REBI, WHAT do you know?" my mother asked as Michel and Cindy pulled up in the new Jeep. "I do all the work and Michel ends up with a rich wife with houses everywhere."

Rebi gave my mother a sympathetic look and hugged her good-bye. She was great with my mother, even though my mother often ridiculed her. Once, my mother kicked her out at three a.m. because she was so worried Rebi might have lice—we had just gotten rid of it ourselves, and my mother was convinced all her hair would fall out if she had to treat lice one more time—and even after that Rebi was still willing to sleep over.

Rebi was also still sweet to her even after my mother told her that *Ruth* thought she was a lesbian. I rolled my eyes to let Rebi know that my mother was being a jerk, but I could tell she was hurt.

Rebi was always generous, unfazed, even good-natured when she was corralled into my mother's rabid cleaning frenzies and then berated, at times, for being "pathetic." I would hover nearby, mopping the kitchen or folding clothes, while my mother teased her about her sweeping technique, torn between raw shame and an unnerving feeling of camaraderie with my mother.

I noticed this same feeling when my mother's depressive, always hungry friend, Dita, picked at things in the fridge. My mother would suddenly scream, "Oh, Dita, just take out the roast and eat it, for God's sake!" or "I can't take it anymore, Dita! That constant chewing! You've got to go. My nerves are on edge."

I would tell my mother, afterward, that she had been too mean to Dita, yet while it was happening, I saw Dita through my mother's eyes—I saw her skinny shoulders hunched over the roast, and the sound of her smacking lips began to wear on my nerves as well until

I, too, had the urge to yell, "Next time eat dinner before you stop by without calling!" and kick the door shut behind her.

"Michel really knows how to pick 'em, huh?" my mother continued.

I reminded her that Cindy wasn't that rich and us kids being away was a great opportunity for her to get some work done.

"He always had to have the best of everything," she said, directing her speech to Rebi. "We'd be totally broke, but he would only buy cashmere sweaters. He said everything else itched his skin. He said his mother always bought him cashmere . . . Well, let's see how long Cindy will last. Have fun, girls!" she said with fake cheer as we got into the car.

"Lub you, Mom!" Gaby called out from the Jeep window. I was bringing her along for the first time.

From the passenger seat, Cindy waved to my mother and smiled sweetly. I was so grateful for her ability to pretend nothing bad was happening.

There was nothing worse to me than when a person tried to discuss my mother's behavior with me.

My mother smiled back at Cindy—the kind of smile she used for pictures—wide and even, her pointy eyeteeth displayed.

The week before, when Michel dropped us off on Sunday, my mother ran out to the Jeep and yelled something at him as he was driving away. He made an aggressive U-turn on Twenty-third Street, pulled back up in front of the hotel without completely stopping, yelled *fuck you*, and then screeched off again.

After he disappeared around the corner, she said, "See? He must be using again or he wouldn't have just acted so crazy."

"My mom got really cuckoo last week . . . *as usual, ha ha!*" I said as we pulled away.

Gaby said, "Yeah, she's cwazy sometimes, wight, Webi?"

"Right," Rebi said, putting her arm around Gaby.

Everyone laughed. Relief.

I had learned to preempt anyone's reaction to my mother. I wanted it to be known that I knew what they thought, and I would prefer if they said nothing about it at all. I could make jokes about her, but I bristled when anyone else did.

I draped my leg over Rebi; she leaned back and closed her eyes; Gaby put her head in my lap. We were on our way to an alternate universe of Cindy's creation, a magical land of kitsch and comfort where we miraculously functioned smoothly—a reprieve, for a time, from what lived underneath.

As we drove toward the West Side Highway I looked out the rear window and watched my mother standing under the Chelsea awning, hands on her hips, getting smaller and smaller.

Now

I'm clearing the mail and the video equipment from our dining room table, spreading a pink tablecloth, filling a huge carved-wood bowl with fruit, and decorating the table with candles, spruce branches, and holly to create a Christmas mise-en-scène.

Gaby is trying to cajole Miko off the screen to make a pie with Rosy. Instead, Miko grabs a Nerf gun and starts shooting Lewis. I'm tense because Gaby's kids are not allowed screens and guns.

"Mom, why does your face look like this?" Miko asks, mocking me by contorting his own face to look like he's disgusted by something.

"Sometimes I want to walk around with a paper bag over my head," I say to Gaby.

Mom walks through and says, "I don't know how you two do it all, you poor things."

You poor thing.

Gaby and I look at each other.

You poor thing means we are martyred. *You poor things* means she thinks we are like her. *You poor things* means she thinks I'm saddled with a lazy bastard husband, or that Lui is a slut, or that Miko is spoiled. *You poor things* means she wants to commiserate with us about how much work we have to do. We will not commiserate! This is life, bitch! You couldn't handle it, but we can! Look at us doing it all!

Most of this Christmas prep is for Cindy. I yearn to return her generosity and re-create in some way the bounty she has always offered us—at least in hearth and home—because we could never repay all her financial help. But we have to remember not to be too good to her in front of Mom. This would leave our behavior toward Mom bare and beating on the floor like a cold heart she can't ignore.

Over the years Cindy has often hosted Christmas for Gaby and me and our kids. Gaby and I have shared some guilt over not including Mom—it would be too much, too overwhelming to moderate Mom's reactions to the perfect splendor that Cindy orchestrates over the holidays—so we have never really described Cindy's domestic mastery to Mom.

Other than our wedding and some graduations, this will be the first time Cindy and Viva have been under the same roof together.

Cindy is currently pulling from the trunk of her Tesla an obscene—but thoroughly appreciated—number of presents.

She is, as always, impossibly youthful looking with pale skin and fine features. Her grayish-blue eyes have a tender birdlike quality. Birds are her favorite creatures. After Birdie died, she adopted her parrot—Mr. Frida—and has had him for more than thirty years. Her hairstyle often changes—today it's long and blond with blunt bangs. She is wearing a fashion-forward ensemble: platform sneakers, an oversize Prada fanny pack in fluorescent orange, and a modern take on an oversize prairie dress. She is petite and almost disappears behind the pile of presents she is holding as she walks toward the house.

We all get giddy over one another and all the presents and finally settle in the kitchen. Cindy has also brought a case of wine and a fifties-style gingerbread house she made herself.

I'm terribly nervous. Beyond their twenty-year age difference, the two women are a striking contrast next to each other, though neither one of them seems particularly insecure when faced with the other.

Mom is less confrontational; maybe she is placated by Cindy's generous deference to her.

"Can you believe all this work Alex did?" my mother says to Cindy as Gaby pours us all some wine.

Gaby and I take a sip and say, with our eyes, this is going well so far.

"I mean both Gaby and Alex are domestic goddesses!" my mother says.

"They learned from the best!" Cindy says.

"I'm a total slob," my mother says.

"Look, Mom," Gaby says, "Cindy is a gingerbread craftswoman just like you used to be."

"I see!" Mom says, looking at Cindy's house. "Verrryyy good, Cindy!"

Cindy and Viva seem downright cozy with each other. Their bonding subject quickly switches from gingerbread to Michel's fuckery.

Over the years, in the rare moments we have talked about him, I have never begrudged Cindy her Michel resentment. Usually I try to throw in some little snarky snippets here and there about his serial relationships with women under thirty-five just so it doesn't seem as though I am on his "side," or like I'm squirreling away information, and Cindy kindly never searches me for more details.

I'm briefly tempted to tell Cindy and Viva about how, as they speak, I'm currently fielding text messages from his sweet but apparently insane twenty-nine-year-old girlfriend, whom he has recently ghosted, and who has devolved into an obsessed, sobbing stalker who regularly laments—to me—about her aborted "Auder child." But I do not let the women in on this tidbit because the fact that I actually take her calls makes me look worse than my father, so I try to casually distance myself from the conversation while I prepare Christmas Eve dinner.

Cindy is now reminding Viva about how she helped Michel get clean by putting him through three rehabs, financially supporting him for the entirety of their marriage, and then, after he left her for a younger woman, she had to pay him alimony for seven more years.

Mom hoots and howls over this.

"Oh, he was just so irresponsible!" Mom is saying. "He has always done that! Just dumped things when he got sick of them. Cindy, listen: in Europe he would rent cars, total them, and then just dump them on the side of the road!"

"What an asshole," Cindy says, gleefully.

"I'm going to bring the kids to the trampoline," Gaby says, gesturing for me to join her. I don't follow her. I have some kind of sick need to hear more.

Nick passes through the kitchen with two bags full of dirty laundry and heads down to the basement.

"And of course as you well know, Cindy—and I tried to warn you—he is a complete and utter gigolo. He rented another apartment in the Chelsea just to fuck other women."

"Are you kidding?" Cindy says.

"No!"

"What a cocksucker."

"But, Cindy. How could you have knowingly married a junkie?!"

OK, there's the bitchiness, I think. *He may have been a heroin addict, but at least he wasn't a cunt from hell.*

"It was really stupid of me, I guess," Cindy says with a tone of bitter acceptance.

"So, Mom, you've only ever been with excellent men?" I counter.

"Ha!" my mother says, letting me have that.

My mother goes into the usual: men are weak, men are lazy, men are pathetic, men are babies, men always abandon you, men exploit you, men are violent.

And what are you, Mom? A sacrificial lamb? An exploited saint? A peacekeeper?

"Nick is an amazing father, though," Cindy says.

I'm dying to look at my mother's face. Before she has a chance to say anything, Nick comes back up from the basement with a bag of clean laundry and winks at me.

"Did someone call my name?" he says.

"No, Nick," my mother says.

"Nick" comes out sounding like she wanted to say: "Scum of the earth." She looks at Cindy with a wry smile and adds: "We were just talking about how all men are useless . . . except, of course, for you, *Nick.*" And here she says *Nick* with saccharine sweetness.

My back is to them, and I want to bash her over the head with the cast-iron pan I'm using to sauté onions.

"If it weren't for me, you'd have no dairy," Nick says as he picks up the butter and half-and-half I left out earlier and sticks them in the fridge.

My mother and Cindy don't know what he's talking about, so they ignore him.

But I do. He thinks I never put the dairy back in the fridge. I'd normally roll my eyes and say, "And if it weren't for me, you'd be drooling in a corner," but I would never ever say anything remotely derogatory toward Nick in front of my mother. She would pounce on it. She would lap up my resentment like a starving dog. God, she would love it. I've never done it. For twenty-five years I've never said a single even slightly off-kilter word about Nick in front of my mother.

But when my mother is not physically around—when her actual voice is absent—wicked words come cascading into my skull: *lazy fuck, how dare you nag at me, blah blah, when I do all the cooking blah blah blah, you'd be fumbling around looking for the butter in your sock drawer, blah, blah, I could march upstairs right now and shove this butter up your ass while you lounge in bed, blah, blah, blah.*

They say your ve̶r̶ ⌗first thoughts are the internalized dialogue of the mother figure (whoever raised you). Your first words were you mimicking what you heard around you; then one day that person shushed you, and you turned the words inward, and they became thoughts. So your thoughts are not your own.

OK, I've got to get out of this kitchen.

I find Gaby on the trampoline with the kids.

"Everything OK?" she asks nervously.

"Oh yeah, just the usual Koo Koo Roo." (Nick gave my mother this code name—it's her favorite fast-food chain. *His* mother's code name is another of my mother's favorites: El Pollo Loco.)

We lie next to each other on the trampoline, letting the kids plop on us. Gaby looks at me and lifts an eyebrow. Her eyebrow is a rune, speaking what can't be said.

Chapter 16

Stolen Time

R ebi and I were officially teenagers, but nothing had changed. We kept getting taller while adding no flesh. We were still waiting for blood and boobs.

Every morning Denise-the-operator gave us our wake-up call. My mother would answer the shrill Chelsea ring with a quick, sleepy "Thanks," and then would ask me if I wanted her to make me breakfast.

I always encouraged her to stay in bed because on the mornings when she did get up along with me, the way she slinked around the apartment in her flannel nightgown, straining coffee with an old sock and making moaning sounds, irritated me. And if I had told her that I actually preferred to eat breakfast at the Squat, where Eva would serve us frothy hot chocolate in a bowl, I knew she would insist on making me something herself. But if I acted like I was doing her a favor by not making her get up out of bed—then she would agree to ignore me and I would have the quiet morning to myself while she and Gaby slept.

I needed this time to relentlessly smooth down my curly hair with mousse. It was a lost cause, though, because even when I slept with a hat on, by the time I checked myself out in the bathroom mirror at school my hair had poofed out again.

In math class I would stare at the back of Sarah Fab's head, trying to figure out how she got her hair so smooth and shiny with two barrettes on either side, holding it away from her heart-shaped face like an open curtain.

When my mother asked why I was wearing a hat to bed, and I complained about my hair, she told me the story of how, when she was a kid, a girl was so jealous of her ringlets that she persuaded her mother to iron them out, and from then on her hair was frizzy and ruined. Even the jealous girl's mother said, "What happened to Sue's gorgeous hair?!" Then, she said, so many years later, when she was famous, her frizzy hair was a huge sensation and everyone tried to copy it, even Madonna.

"So that Sarah Fab girl is probably a real bore."

I wasn't convinced.

Before I left the apartment I applied black eyeliner to the inside rims of my lower lids. Sometimes, on my way out the door, my mother might get up to say goodbye and take my chin in her hand and hold my face up close to hers, and say, as though I had slashed my face with a razor, "Oh, honey, why are you wearing so much makeup to school?"

"It's just eyeliner and mascara."

"I don't think that's appropriate. You're barely fourteen, for God's sake."

"It's nothing, *God*."

"Honey, do you know how much time I used to waste putting on makeup? I mean I put *liquid* eyeliner on while I was in Morocco, for God's sake! You're so young and beautiful! You'll realize that when you're old. You'll realize that you never needed makeup. When you're young, you always look the best *totally natural . . .*"

I could never be sure what her reaction to things would be. One week she might be totally laissez-faire about something, and the next week she'd be enforcing rules and regulations. So I wasn't surprised when one morning she suddenly announced: "I forbid you to wear that black eyeliner to school anymore."

"Fine," I said, deadpan, planning to apply the liner in the school bathroom.

She had begun to tell her friends things on the phone that she really wanted me to hear. Sometimes I couldn't care less, but other times, the words felt like literal stab wounds.

"She's been wearing it to school *every* day. I didn't notice at first because she was *racing* over to Eva's—the *saint*. So trashy. I think she's too young. I mean she doesn't even have tits, for Christ's sake."

As I started to walk out the door, she would yell, "Wait! Be very careful! Don't go to that donut place on the corner—they might all have AIDS! You can get it from saliva. *Saliva!*"

"OK, don't worry," I would say, humoring her in order to get out the door.

When I arrived at the Squat, I'd often have to play a song on the buzzer to wake Eva and Rebecca on the fourth floor. Once I got into the building, I'd climb up the stairs and sit on the side of Rebi's bed while she quickly changed under the covers, next to the kerosene heater. We could see our breath on the coldest winter days. Rebi put thick tights underneath her velvet pants to lend her legs a little more bulk because she worried that she looked too thin.

Eva would make us soft-boiled eggs and pack Rebi's lunch with Hungarian fare, like liver pâté on thick pumpernickel bread with cucumber slices and paprika, which I would later encourage her to throw out so I could buy us both lunch at Blimpie's or Mr. Pizza with the cash I had grabbed from the top drawer. It was a wicked act, throwing away the food that Eva had procured by carefully saving money, biking to the Lower East Side to get cheap spices and Hungarian ingredients, and biking the special foods back home from sacks hanging off her arms.

ON THE WEEKENDS Rebi and I brought Gaby to Eighth Street in the stroller, where we hung out with friends on the corner and bought rubber bracelets at Postermat.

Sometimes we would take Gaby to the indoor McDonald's playground, climb up a little ladder and cram our tall bodies inside the giant plastic hamburger, while Gaby ran around with other toddlers. While she was distracted by the other kids, we would space out inside the filthy burger, our bodies bent and folded awkwardly to accommodate the round shape, stare out the jail-cell bars between the two buns, slurp vanilla milkshakes, and eat the little rectangular apple pies.

Rebi and I alternated where we were going to sleep on weekends and sometimes weekday nights. I would rather have been in the freezing Squat—huddled under the covers with Rebi, waiting for the theater to empty out so we could scavenge for spare change to buy candy at Lamstons—than hang out with Rebi in my own warm apartment with easily accessible cash in the top drawer. At my place, we had to sardine our lanky, oversize bodies into the narrow top bunk, scraping our skin all night on the sharp paint, and deal with my mother at our feet.

Certain mornings, when we knew we couldn't face the dismal walk to school and the ensuing doldrums that would unfold, we kissed Eva goodbye, made a quick stop at Lamstons for Charleston Chews, frosted pink wet *n* wild lipstick, and Merit cigarettes, and instead of walking down Eighth Avenue to Seventeenth Street, we turned left on Twenty-second Street and walked through the parking lot behind the Squat. There the parking attendant gave us a wink when we used the hood of a parked car to reach the last rung of the fire escape where we hoisted ourselves up and began to climb the ladder. We passed the second floor windows where Pisti was in his white underwear, tangled up in the sheets, sound asleep. We passed the third floor windows where we saw Agnes naked, stretching, her long black hair spilling out on the floor. We passed the fourth floor windows where Eva had hung a dark velvet curtain, and then we scrambled over the lip of the roof.

The rooftops were connected all the way to the corner of Twenty-third and Eighth Avenue. We made our way to the end of the buildings—jumping down onto the roofs when they didn't meet up flush. We dangled our legs over the edge of the last building while we smoked, spit down to the sidewalk, and surveyed the street scene down below. Men in leather bombers and tight jeans, old women with rounded backs pushing grocery carts, drunk men swaying from curb to curb, someone nodding out against the garbage bin, a bike with a boom box strapped to the side playing the Sugarhill Gang.

"What the fuck?!" some people would yell out after we spit, looking up and trying to figure out what had landed on their heads.

When it was too cold out, we sheltered in the glass house—a strange little structure on the roof that was sometimes empty, but other times was, unpredictably, the temporary bedroom of a bearded homeless-seeming man with a heavy accent, who we assumed was a friend of the Squat's visiting from out of town, but might have been actually homeless, or maybe he was the undercover CIA or KGB agent who, they would discover, was sent to spy on them. The "house" had a ladder that led up to a loft platform with a mattress under a glass ceiling. In the summertime it was an oven, but in cold weather—if the sun was out—it was the perfect shelter. We would lie next to each other on the old mattress, empty candy wrappers scattered around, our blood quickened by sugar, and we would stare up at the white clouds passing across the glass, waiting for a sign, a message from the sky telling us who would ravish us and how soon.

For lunch, we climbed all the way back down the building and ate at the Ritz Diner, my mother's favorite. We smoked a cigarette when we were finished with our mashed potatoes and turkey gravy, scanning the sidewalk from inside the diner, freezing with terror when we thought we had seen my mother's frizzy hair pass by.

If the goat from the play *Pig Child Fire!* was around, we might sneak it out for a walk on a leash, making sure to stay hidden in the gardens behind the apartment buildings on another block.

"Yo, that's a goat!" some guy would call out and we would laugh, self-aware of the uncanny image—two extraordinarily tall kids wearing velvet pants and walking a hoofed creature on Eighth Avenue.

ONE DAY, when we crested the top of the fire escape, Eva was waiting for us on the roof. "Playing hooky, huh?" she yelled, but she also laughed. She forced us to come inside to warm up and allowed us to squander the rest of the day locked in a fourth floor bedroom. She even brought us snacks. While we ate we listened to Bob Dylan.

"Listen," Rebi said, quoting, "'But she breaks just like a little girl . . .'" Rebi frowned. "I love him but I just think it's weird. I think he's fucked up—she *breaks* like a little girl?"

We rewound the tape and listened again.

Suddenly something was terribly wrong.

My mother's voice was echoing through the building.

The walls vibrated and my vision blurred. I could hear Eva trying to calm her, but her voice got closer, louder.

"You're living with a bunch of junkies, Eva, face it! It's pathetic! I don't want my daughter around this! I want to be *told* when she's skipping school. How do you think I felt when I found out she wasn't there? You just want everyone to love you and you'll do anything, *anything* not to rustle their feathers!"

It was all wrong to see her inside the Squat; just like the way Eva didn't fit in our apartment, my mother was out of her element, but the tone of her voice seemed to be linked to my cells.

I SOON DISCOVERED that pretending to be at ballet was the perfect ruse for buying myself time at the Squat. If my mother believed I was *working* at ballet, honing my talent—which was meager according to the old hags at the school—I could escape her fury.

Usually I would hang out at the Squat for an hour before I had to get the Eighth Avenue bus uptown for class. One afternoon I missed the bus and went back to the Squat, skipping class.

The next afternoon I found myself still standing in the vestibule between the front door and the theater door instead of waiting for the bus on the corner. After a minute of staring straight ahead, I walked back up to the fourth floor and told Rebi that I wasn't going. Soon I stopped going to class entirely. It felt reckless and thrilling.

When the stolen time entered my bloodstream, I pleasantly tuned out, edges blurred, drifting on a raft in the middle of nowhere, my hand dipped in the water. But as the clock ticked toward evening, my freedom was more precarious; guilt and dread began to nip at my fingers, at first gently, then eating ribbons of flesh.

I told myself every week that I would not do it again, but every week, as class time drew closer and closer, I simply remained on the raft with Rebi and some other Squat kids, watching TV and entering our imaginary worlds for the two-hour span that my pliés and chassés were accounted for in my mother's imagination.

I was addicted.

For the next three months, I would arrive home at around seven p.m. and tell my mother about the ballet class I hadn't actually been to.

I got better at lying to her. When she thought she was the sacrificial one, that's when I was more vulnerable to her moods. But when I got home, supposedly exhausted from ballet class, with a load of homework, I always had the upper hand.

"Honey, you must be so tired," she would say. "How was class?"

"*Hard*," I would say, turning on the television and opening my schoolbooks.

"You must be exhausted. I'm worried about subway shootings. I think you should take the bus from now on. Please."

I made some calculations and realized that she had assumed I had been taking the subway this whole time. The subway was faster. So now, if she thought I had switched to the bus, she would expect me home even later.

"Good idea," I said.

Each time I had to leave the Squat to return home, I grasped onto the edges of the threshold, not wanting to transition at all. This drove Rebi crazy because it was a literal grasping—we would be sprawling on a mattress on the floor, bingeing on one TV show after another—*Diff'rent Strokes, The Facts of Life, Charles in*

Charge—and Rebi would get up to do something, anything—go pee—and I would seize one of her legs, wrap myself around it, dropping into my full dead body weight.

The stolen time spread itself out like a clingy web; I was suspended at its center, guilt and worry lurking along the periphery.

"Five more minutes!" I would beg her to stay, to not move, and she would become genuinely upset. It was the only time she would ever yell at me. She told me very clearly that she absolutely hated it when I held her down like that, yet I still thought I could charm her into staying put, that my desperation would be compelling, that she would take pity on me.

It never worked. Eventually I had to leave.

As I walked home, I prepared myself, mentally, for the charade.

I hit the gold elevator button with the heel of my hand and used the key to scratch out the name *Sid* and replace it with *Alex*.

ONE AFTERNOON WHEN I was supposed to be at ballet, Rebi and I were listening to the radio when George Michael's "Everything She Wants" came on.

"Jesus, what a selfish asshole! Now you tell me that you're having *my* baby?!" Rebi yelled at our boom box.

"Yeah, I'm so sure *his* back will break—what a dick!"

"One step further?! He's so threatening!"

"Yeah, dude, *she's* the pregnant one!"

"Dinner!" Eva yelled up the stairwell.

The phone rang as I sat at one of the round café tables, eating Eva's delicious food.

I immediately knew it was my mother—her anger traveling from number 710 through the phone wires had somehow made the ring sound different. Eszter answered and now she approached me with a worried look on her face. I looked at the big kitchen clock. It had ticked past the time I should have been home from the bus after ballet.

Fuck, I had lost track.

"Alex—you better talk to your mom," Eszter said, sounding grave.

I entered the little phone stall and put my ear to the receiver. I heard breathing.

"Mom?"

A pause.

"I thought you were dead. The police are on their way to the hotel."

Prickly zips and zaps fired under my skin and knocked me out of my body. I left, zombie-walking down the half block. As I entered the Chelsea, Merle and Stanley may have been calling my name but I wouldn't have known.

I stood in front of the apartment door, laying my hand on it and waiting—like Ellen Burstyn in *Resurrection*—trying to feel what disease lurked on the other side. The door throbbed. I stared at it until I had devised a plan.

When I opened it, the air was still.

"I'm in here," she called out with an unnerving depth and calmness to her voice.

She was lying in bed, having taken the collapse approach.

"For two months I've been paying for those classes and you haven't even been there. *Two months*. Can you imagine what I thought when I frantically called to see why you were so late? I thought you were dead. *Dead*."

My plan was for her to think she had power over me again, so I went with full disclosure, complete vulnerability. I laid myself at her feet, cried, begged for forgiveness, acknowledged the money wasted, appealed to her loathing of provinciality by describing the uptight teachers who were blind to my talents.

It worked.

We were soon lying in bed together, me crying for forgiveness, her offering it with affection. "Of course I'll still trust you. I just don't understand why you lied. Don't worry. I love you, honey. You're overworked . . ."

It went on like that while she hugged me and sort of jerked me in closer every now and then, the way she did when she was trying to reassure me. I knew if I allowed for the *illusion* of the secret-free state, I would still be able to keep secrets.

Yet she remained suspicious.

For the next few months, when I returned home from actual ballet class, she would raise her eyebrows when she asked me about the class. In order to act natural and to create the sense of ease that truth telling produces, I had to work harder than I had anticipated.

When I demonstrated a step we had learned in class, she laughed and said, "You just made that up!" The more defensive I became, the more disingenuous I seemed, even though I had indeed just been to class.

"Call the school if you want and ask them if I was there! I don't care what you think!" I finally yelled one afternoon.

She was standing with her hands on her hips, watching me. With a weary, condescending tone, she said, "I *believe* you, honey. Go ahead, show me the steps."

Instead, I stormed into the other room.

Chapter 17

G-Spot

Rebi and I had a vicious fight over who had cherry pits or peach pits for tits and which one of us had one more straggly pubic hair than the other.

Our desires were mounting, but boys would have nothing to do with us, so I often fantasized about men. My desire could be specific, like wanting mouth on mouth contact, but often it was more abstract, like the yearning for unfettered psychic space. At Rebi's we were free, or at least I felt free to explore my fantasies.

When there was no current production, the Squat turned into a nightclub where Sun Ra played live shows, and Vincent Gallo hosted a film night screening hard-to-see movies like *Cuksucker Blues*. During these nights Rebi and I lived in our own shared fantasy worlds, secretly lusting over Gallo's sinister good looks when he passed us in the hall.

We were inspired, vicariously, by our sexual mentors—Boris (Rebi's older sister) and Eszter—dark humored, Eastern European versions of Betty and Veronica—Eszter the brunette, Boris the blonde. They were just a few years older than us, yet they seemed like fully developed women with sexy older lovers.

Eszter, at sixteen, had already dated the artist Jean-Michel Basquiat, who was six years older than her. I had no idea there was even a discrepancy in their age. They just seemed cool together, and for me the coolness blurred their ages. Then she was with Stephen, a talkative, charming, disheveled friend of Jean-Michel's. Boris, still a teenager, was with Danny, a beautiful and sad Irish man who must have been in his late twenties. These two mysterious couples would breeze through the Squat on their way to . . . *where*? Rebi and I had no idea. We were late-blooming fourteen-year-olds, swathed in Eva's velvet and corduroy, huddled in a corner playing *Little House on the Prairie* while we lusted after the men.

Rebi was analyzing a Michael Jackson song.

"What an asshole!" she was saying.

"I know," I said.

"*Really* listen to this part . . ." Rebi insisted. Jackson was singing about Billie Jean.

I hit PAUSE, slammed my hand down, and said, "*Claims?* What a jerk—that's what all men say, you know? Oh, you just *claim* it's my kid!"

"I know. *Just a girl?*" Rebi was furious. "I mean they obviously had something together and to call her a *girl* is so fucking condescending."

"Who is so condescending?" Irish Danny asked as he and Boris passed through the room. He was all bedhead and soulful eyes. The couples would sometimes stop and chat with us on their way out to do the mysterious things. They were so mature, so exotic, so brooding, so effortlessly chic!

After they left, we drew anonymous male faces on pieces of paper and tacked the faces up to the loft bed's posts to make out with their ink mouths until the paper dissolved under our slobber. We were also still happily pretending to be surviving on the frigid prairie, mistresses of the Wild West who would somehow find the time to copulate. First, we would make sure the horses were properly tethered, then we would make love to our husbands under the canopy of the covered wagon.

"Wait," Rebi once interrupted as we wrapped our legs around the horsehair pillows. "Would we really do it next to each other in the same wagon?"

"We would do what we need to do to survive," I reassured her.

Just before I was blotted out, the generic stud face I was fantasizing about would transmute into a scruffy-faced Irish Danny, or sometimes more shocking fodder would appear—like Kojak.

Never would my actual love, my classmate Jason Cooney, appear in these orgasmic visions. He was reserved for kissing fantasies. In reality he was going out with Sarah Fab of the straight hair who was everything I would never be. But who did I want actual sex with after all? Jason Cooney's penis appeared in my mind like a blurry Ken doll crotch. I couldn't get off to that. In the visceral part of my fantasies were different cocks and tongues and hands of all the older men I was crushed on: Irish Danny, my French uncle-in-law, Alex P. Keaton, Kojak, and the Fonz.

MAYBE ALL THIS PENT-UP energy was why I had nailed an audition to play a precocious oversexed teen in a coming-of-age movie. In rehearsals for my callback, my mother had cackled with laughter when I seductively whispered the punch line in her ear, which was something like "And that's how you find my G-spot."

It was the first role I had landed on my own and I was overjoyed. I would have an on-set tutor and miss a good chunk of the last bit of eighth grade.

Take that, Sarah Fab.

Gaby, my mother, and I packed for the shoot and boarded the first-class flight to San Diego, where we would be on location for a few weeks.

During the flight, my tutor—required by the board of education— casually suggested to my mother that the G-spot line was inappropriate for a fourteen-year-old to say. When we arrived, hair and makeup gave me a new look for the character—a boy's short haircut.

When I returned to the hotel room, my mother was in a mood— she had been reading the script.

"The lines are obscene, honey. I'm going to talk to the producers."

"Mom, no. That's how my character has to speak—it's the funny part. It's meant to be over the top . . ."

"I don't know. I think they should change the G-spot line— you're too young to be saying that stuff!"

Before we were even in the first rehearsal, the tutor had called the child labor department, and the child labor department said unless the lines were changed, they had to hire an adult, and my mother was arguing with the director.

"Just write different lines! It's ridiculous writing anyway! What? You're so attached to this stupid script that you can't just throw in a new line? Look, I'll do it for you, I'll write a new line right here on the spot . . . Jesus Christ! With Andy we used to just make up all our lines! Andy didn't give a shit about a script! Every good director knows things have to change at the last minute; don't be pathetic! Well, we're going to sue you."

They ended up hiring an eighteen-year-old and paying me the contractual agreement—$10,000—and we packed back up again and left for the San Diego Zoo.

I was devastated. I'd have rather been in the movie for free than get paid to *not* do the part, and now I had to go back to face my peers at IS 70 with a puffball of a haircut and a mouthful of braces.

AROUND THIS TIME is when my mother became fixated on getting a face-lift. It was odd because we had always ridiculed the actresses who had plastic surgery.

My aunt Jeannie knew Ivo Pitanguy, one of the most famous plastic surgeons in the world, and my mother had been wanting to go back to South America to research the Tupamaros for an article she was writing.

Besides being passionately kissed, there was nothing I wanted more than to have the apartment to myself. I was willing to do anything to get her to go, including paying for the trip with the movie money.

"Honey, what do you think I should do, *really*?" she asked.

I weighed my strategy while she paced around the house making calls and trying to decide. This would have to be a delicate maneuver.

"We have the money from the movie, so that takes care of that . . . and this guy is a friend of Jeannie's?" I asked her, trying to sound concerned before I sent her off to get sliced up.

"He's supposed to be the best."

I never knew she didn't like her nose until she started talking about getting a nose job. In the past she had laughed about how

Grandpa thought her nose was too big, and something about how hating women had something to do with his hating her nose.

She had been doing research on what she called Freud's nose obsession—maybe that put the nose job in her mind.

I didn't consider telling her what I really thought—that it was crazy to get a nose job—because I just wanted her out.

I had to have her out.

In my head I ticked off the things that might make me want to persuade her *not* to go: the hell of helping her pack, missing Gaby too much, saving our money, possible disfiguration, she and Gaby getting killed by the revolutionaries.

Helping her pack seemed the most immediately daunting. I looked around the apartment I had just tidied up and thought about how the next day I would get home from school and have to clean it up all over again. I would have to throw the dirty underwear into the hamper; put away her clothes; make the bed; put old issues of the *Post* and *New York Times* in neat piles; throw out the peels, Coke bottles, and coffee-filter socks; wipe the orange juice from the countertops. I would have to ignore the enema bag hanging from the shower curtain rod. That in particular always threw me into a vicious interior rage: *motherfucking shit bag from hell.* She could live with a mess, I couldn't. Really, she couldn't live with a mess either, but she couldn't not make a mess.

"I really think you *need* this," I told her.

"You do?" she asked sincerely.

I knew not to be too insistent. I had to make it seem like:

1. It was her idea.
2. It would be a drag for me to be without her.
3. I would be selflessly letting go of her as a favor.

"Yeah, I do. I think it's important for you to get out of here for a while. You keep saying how much you hate the city."

"But I feel terrible spending all your money."

"It's *our* money, Mom. I don't care at all. Anyway, it's just . . . money. Your sanity is worth more than the money. And it'll be good for your writing."

"Oh, honey, you are so smart. *Really?*" She gave me the lifted eyebrow look—like maybe I was up to something.

"I mean I wish *I* could go too, but I have school. Or . . . I could keep Gaby here, but no, that wouldn't work because I've got to go to school. I'll miss you so much!"

"I shouldn't spend that money, though."

It had to be *her* idea. That way I couldn't be blamed if anything went wrong.

"I really don't care about the money at all. But don't go if you think you shouldn't. You *do* need to get away, though."

My mother was always worried about money, yet we rarely economized. Sometimes we went to McDonald's, or ate frozen Hungry-Man dinners, or put dinner on our tab at the sushi restaurant. When the top drawer was actually empty of cash, my mother would write an article, or call Max Palevsky, or ask Grandpa to send us some cash.

When the money came, we were extravagant: we took cabs to Central Park so my mother could bring her easel, we satisfied cravings for blintzes with black caviar, or we called down to the El Quijote and used an alias and a fake accent to order lobsters, and then asked Jerome to pick up the order for us (we had been banned from the El Quijote after my mother had a fight with the manager and called him a spic).

She began to agonize over what kind of plastic surgery she

should get: just the nose; nose and face; nose, face, and eyes; nose and eyes. I figured the more she had done, the longer she would be away.

"If it will make you feel better—have everything done," I told her.

The packing started. Our apartment looked like the aftermath of a flooded beach town—sunblocks, vitamins, moisturizers, bikinis, rain gear, parkas, snow boots, plastic sandals, sarongs, wool socks, a turned over chair, and straw hats scattered all over the rug.

I was her weather sage, her coach, her gofer. I started to enjoy my different roles because I was no longer worried about her changing her mind—she had actually bought the tickets, and they were on the kitchen table along with a pile of *New York Times Book Reviews*.

She asked my advice in the early morning hours: "Will we be warm enough with just six pairs of wool socks? Will the sun burn through the small straw hat? Perhaps the big old one with the holes was better? Rain boots and snow boots? Snow boots and long underwear? Goggles? Will you really be OK without us? What if Gaby gets impetigo? I'm crazy, aren't I? Tell me the truth. I'm going to have to buy another duffel bag for the blender."

IT WAS SPRING. Our last few months of eighth grade. As the city thawed and buds started popping open, we gave up hope that we might blossom before the summer began. Rebi and I would be going to LaGuardia High School in September. She got in for art and I got in for drama. We would bide our time until then.

Blood did come, but only from my nose. I was sitting in class at IS 70, and a large drop of blood plopped on a white page of my notebook and splattered across the desk. I cupped my hand to my nose and left class. In the bathroom I gathered a wad of toilet paper, but the blood soaked through right away. It was a more profuse nosebleed than usual.

I left school and quickly walked to the Chelsea with the blood seeping through a wad of paper towels. By the time I got to the lobby, the blood was dripping down my chest.

Rather than wait for the elevator, I pushed open the El Quijote doors and slipped into the Chiquita bathroom, risking being seen by the manager.

In the middle of the day only the usual drunks were at the bar. One of them was a woman who looked uncannily like the new Chelsea operator, Bonnie, who looked like she'd stepped out of my favorite John Waters movie, *Female Trouble*.

Once I was safely in the bathroom, I dipped my head down over the sink, and blood slowly poured from my right nostril into the little white basin.

Finally, I was able to stanch the flow enough to get the key from the box and get up to the empty apartment.

I sat on the windowsill for a while and let the quiet drape over me. In the absence of my mother I was left with a sense of nothingness . . . or sadness . . . it was hard to tell. Tears came.

I leaned way out the window—over the childproof bars my mother finally had gotten Stanley to install—and contemplated the alley down below. It had a long thin crack in the concrete from when an old man across the way jumped off the roof and killed himself. I imagined my own body splayed out on the concrete. I would die without having my period and having only ever kissed my cousin Steve.

If I died, my mother might sentence herself to a bedridden life . . . and poor Gaby. No, I had to stay around for Gaby. Without me she would have to deal with my mother on her own. Although she would be so cute at my funeral: "My sistuh was so gweat and funny and pwitty. She helped waise me."

My agents might make a speech. "She was just about to break out," one would say, and then his partner would add, "All the casting directors had seen her shine, had seen her potential."

I dragged a chair into the bathroom. The medicine cabinet above the bathroom sink was the only mirror in the apartment. I often sat on the edge of the sink to get up close and pick my face. If I stood with my back to the door, I could get my chest into the frame. This is how I would check my boob growth. To get a view of my pubic hair (or lack of) from afar I needed a chair to stand on.

As I assessed the situation, I saw she had left the enema bag hanging from the rod and the white tube with the bulbous perforated tip dangled in the air, taunting me. I yanked the contraption down and threw it in the cabinet under the sink. Then I stood before the mirror and cupped my hands over my boobs. Peach pits, still . . . maybe slightly fuller around the sides. I smiled. The braces were unforgiving. From the chair, the pubic hairs looked a little less straggly. I pushed my middle finger up inside myself, pulled it out and examined it: clean.

Motherfucker, I whispered.

I cried in the mirror for a minute.

I could hear Shizo rehearsing in the hall. She lived in the apartment right next to ours; it had pink and aqua paint spilling out from under her doorframe. I opened our door and watched her. She was wearing a tight purple cowboy suit with plastic water guns in the holsters and big red ringlets, probably a wig. She had a heavy Eastern European accent. "*You treat me like . . . shotgun!*" she sang, in a high-pitched voice, and when she said "shotgun," she pulled the water guns from her holster and posed like a cowboy. I smiled and gave her thumbs-up before heading over to our neighbor Sydney's apartment.

Months earlier, in the middle of the night, my mother had banged against the bedroom wall with a stapler to get the couple next door to stop fighting. When they didn't stop, my mother called Bonnie and asked her to ring number 712. When they answered, she said, "This is Viva next door and I can't take it anymore! You've got to stop fighting! I'm a nursing mother!"

There was a pause on the other end. Sydney had a slight southern accent. She said, "*Oh my God.* You're Viva Superstar?! I've always loved you . . . I'm so, so sorry about the noise. I met Gaby in the elevator and I'd love to babysit!"

The next day she came over to watch Gaby for a couple of hours, and we all became friends.

Sydney was in her early twenties, with Jean Seberg hair, and she wore red lipstick, torn Levi's, a perfect white T, and Doc Martens. She was my new style mentor.

Her apartment was a single room with a little sink bolted to the wall. The toilet and shower were out in the communal hall. When I walked in, Sydney handed me the phone. I asked Bonnie for room number 708.

We could hear Shizo's phone ringing down the hall.

"Allo?" she said.

"You suck, *Shit-zo*, you'll never be famous," I growled into the phone. Sydney egged me on, gesturing to keep at it. "This is the Crunch," I mumbled. I was pretending to be the lead singer of a rival band who lived and practiced on the floor below us.

I had to keep my voice down because it was possible Shizo could hear our voices coming from inside the apartment.

"Yeah?" she said into the phone, "Vell, *Crunch*, you stink vorse zan garbage; it hurting my ears to hear you practice."

I slammed the phone down, and Sydney and I fell to the bed, cracking up.

Meanwhile, my mother was somewhere in Brazil recovering from surgery: a shaving down of the famous nose her father hated, a slice along the ears to pull the excess forty-six-year-old skin more taut around the cheeks and jawline, slivers cut into the eyelids to erase time.

Chapter 18

The River

G aby was about to run out the dining room doors to the front porch when Grandpa grabbed her by the collar and held her up to the sunlight as if to inspect her closer. He mumbled: "Dark skin, eh? There now, let's see those eyes. Oh, hell! Ha! Cute little tyke, though. Not as dark as Jeannie's kids, huh? Those tykes are real little spics, heh?"

There was that word my mother had called the El Quijote manager.

I cringed.

I knew Grandpa had a fixation on people's origins. And my mother and I had both said to each other that he was racist. But as different as she was from him, I was discovering that my mother was still influenced by his prejudices. She had told Grandpa that she suspected Anthony was from Puerto Rico, not Spain—this, I was deducing, was meant to be a put-down, though I wasn't sure why. Or maybe it was Grandpa who thought it was better to be from Spain, and she was trying to irk him.

"Gwampa, let go!" Gaby squealed.

He put her down and she ran off to find all the little cousins.

It was the summer of 1985. I was fourteen, Gaby was three. She had returned from Brazil with wild hair and a lot more things to say.

When I first saw my mother after the surgery, I thought her nose looked almost the same as it had before, nothing like those turned up noses we ridiculed on *Knots Landing*. It still had the original overall shape, only smaller, which was unsettling. She had asked if I thought she looked younger. I had never thought she looked old, so I said, "You look rested!"

Summer in the city, in our apartment, was hot and stuffy, so we had decided to head to the River. We wanted Gaby to be able to run around with her cousins.

Although no one seemed to remember the fight where my mother and grandfather both ended up at the hospital—or at least they pretended not to—I arrived on guard.

Grandpa's eyes wandered to my breasts and then to my hips. He gripped my shoulders. "Don't hunch now. The Hoffmanns have tall genes, see? And . . . and it's Mother's side that's got the hunch—the McNicholas side, see? See her all hunched? Never listened. Oh, Grandma McNicholas was one hell of a hunchback." He laughed and laughed at the thought of her hunchback. "You watch what you eat now, don't you? I can see that. Nice and slim."

"I'm the hunchback of Notre Dame!" I said as I did a Quasimodo shtick to escape from him and ran down to the dock.

I was wearing an ankle-length tight, black stretchy tube skirt with purple high-top sneakers, a deep V-neck slouchy sweater, a couple of inches' worth of black rubber bracelets on my left wrist interspersed with bright colored metal bracelets studded with rhinestones, and a spirally purple plastic choker; I wanted to repre-

sent New York City and show off how sophisticated I was compared
to my cousins from Los Angeles. But secretly, really, I wanted to
impress Steve.

Oh my God, Allie's here!" my aunts squealed.

Marybeth felt me up and said, "She's got tiny little boobs!
Honey, let's go to Alex Bay to get a training bra."

"You look just like your father . . . Oh! I can't believe it—*just
like him.*"

"So statuesque."

"Remember when you came to Argentina, huh? Huh, my little
Allie Pooh?" Jeannie gritted her teeth like she did when she was
holding a baby and squeezed me. "And now you're all grown up."

"Honey, we've got to buy you some new shoes . . ."

"Would you like that, Alskins?"

"More feminine—some sweet flats?"

"Yes, let's get me a *Little House on the Prairie* dress too," I said
sarcastically.

"Do you have a boyfriend, honey?"

I looked around to see who was listening. Steve was in the water
doing pull-ups on the diving board. Every time he lifted himself up
the water dripped from his flexing muscles. He hoisted himself
onto the diving board, and my eyes were drawn to the indents on
either side of his pelvis forming a path to a hairy line that disappeared under the waistband of his trunks.

"Let's get in the raft," he said to me.

We climbed into the rubber yellow raft and right before we
pushed off, Franny yelled, "Wait for me!" and squeezed in between us.

As we drifted away, I watched the aunts surround Gaby, oohing
and aahing over how cute she was. Then they surrounded my

mother to check out the work she had done on her face. I could see her wincing, pointing to her nose, talking about the wind and how the slightest breeze on her nose was excruciating. Gaby and the little cousins were trying to pierce a live worm with a fishing hook. I heard my mother saying the surgery was more painful than childbirth.

"Do you have your period?" Franny asked. I glanced back at the dock to make sure my mother couldn't hear.

"Yeah," I said.

"And a boyfriend?" Steve asked.

"Yeah." The details of my imaginary love life came so easily that I started to believe it myself. "His name is *Jason Cooney.*"

Franny was impressed. "Have you had sex yet?" she asked.

"Not yet," I said. "But soon."

Steve said he had a girlfriend.

"They had sex," Franny added.

I kept a straight face but secretly burned with jealousy.

As the summer passed, I found myself lovesick and directionless when Steve abandoned me for sports. I occupied myself by orchestrating games with the little cousins that always had something to do with getting naked and shocking Grandpa and making him blame the aunts or at least think they were bad mothers.

One time I talked the little kids into dressing up in pink chiffon curtain material from the bureau at the top of the stairs. Every summer I loved to rediscover what was in the bureau—left from the summers before.

"It's time for Curtain Church," I said. "Grandpa will be very happy if he knows you all became nuns and priests today," I told them.

"You're wrong."

"Not me."

"I will," Gaby said.

"But *you* can't make church."

"Yes she can, she my sistuh!"

"Everyone take off your clothes," I said.

I wrapped some more of the material around bare torsos so the extra chiffon draped down their backs and onto the floor. For chalices we used Grandpa's German beer mugs decorated with little ceramic fräuleins on the handles. I put some chips in a mug and sent them down to Grandpa, who was in the TV den. Gaby led the way and stood in front of Grandpa. I spied on them from the window on the lower stairs landing.

"Take some Communion, Gwandpa, or you'll go to hell!" she said.

He looked so angry it made me a little nervous that he might hit Gaby. I had been hoping one of the other cousins would be the leader—so we wouldn't be associated with these antics—but Gaby was proving to be a formidable accomplice. Luckily, she ran away before Grandpa got to her.

Grandpa never suspected I was behind these things. He still thought I was a "good girl." I even pretended to love church, and as boring as it was, on some level this was true. I loved it because we were all forced to be together. No sports allowed. We got to travel in Grandpa's big black limo that he drove himself, which I thought was ridiculously funny. Not to mention, it was Frog Church.

We called it Frog Church because the priest collected piles and piles of stuffed frogs, frog statues, and frog figurines. People sent him frogs, nobody knew why. The frogs had their own altar; there were so many that they spilled out into the pews. Big blow-up frogs, tiny clay frogs, velvet frogs, and plastic frogs with gold halos.

On Frog Church mornings, Grandpa would wake up before the rest of us, hide the boat keys, lock Soot, his nasty dog, on the kitchen porch, nervously wander from room to room counting heads, and call those family members who were not on the island to make sure they were on their way to church in their own towns and cities.

I flitted around from room to room following the action, keeping mental tabs on who was going where and what Grandpa was tuned into or not tuned into. I might even drop him a hint if I suspected that Marybeth, for example, was attempting to take the boat out instead of going to church. I'd casually pass him, and just loud enough for him to hear I'd say something like: "MB found the boat keys."

"Where . . . Marybeth? Where are you going?" Grandpa spit when he found her quietly opening the screen doors to the big porch.

"Nowhere, Dad. I just wanted to get something I left on the dock."

He looked back at some kids following Marybeth. "Steve and Alexandra, you come in the car with me, now, we're going to be late. Come on now, into the car."

When we arrived, Grandpa tried to lead us in a line to the back pews, but my cousins ran wildly around the church. There were so many cousins now, he had no control. He clenched his fists. Grandma's cleats went *click, click, click* down the aisle. She had worn her golf shoes instead of her pumps. She was starting to lose her marbles, some of the sisters said.

Grandpa said the sound was better in the back, but we all knew he just wanted to hide Marybeth and Mo when they opened their shirts to nurse their babies and toddlers. When Mo pulled out her boob, Grandpa looked furious and started gnawing on his lower lip.

None of us children knew the prayers by heart, so when the time came to pray aloud I made up my own prayers—*please let my mother be happy, please let a boy like me, please let me get those Gloria Vanderbilt jeans.*

Oliver became exasperated with all the standing, sitting, and kneeling, and blurted, "Why do we come here?! All we do is up down God, up down God!"

That's true, I thought, silently laughing.

Grandma looked like she wanted to hit him over the head with the bible.

When it came time to receive Communion, Grandpa grabbed me by the arm—hard—and pulled me close.

"Did you have your First Communion?" he spat into my ear.

I nodded my head.

"Where?" he asked.

"Umm . . . ," I stammered.

My mother appeared and put her hand on my shoulder. "St. Francis, Dad," she said, winking at me.

Grandpa grunted and let go of my sleeve.

I let the priest lay the Eucharist on my outstretched tongue doggy style, as I called it, rather than in the palm of my hands.

After Mass was over I gestured for the little kids to go ahead and run into the frog room, where they writhed around in the pile of stuffed frogs like they were possessed.

GRANDPA THOUGHT I was a good girl until the day he caught me standing on the patch of no-man's-land between the shed and the main house, aiming my middle finger up toward the kitchen, pumping it hard, jutting my ass out, while I mouthed the words *fuck you.* I was mad because he and Uncle Terry told me and Franny that we were lazy good-for-nothings and forced us to haul out some stinky garbage.

When I got back up to the main house, Grandpa cornered me in the dining room and said, "What was that you were doing down there, huh?"

"What was what?"

"That gesture, young lady. With your finger."

"I was dancing . . . is that what you mean? When I was dancing for you, Grandpa?"

STEVE HAD BEEN giving me lessons on how to French-kiss without my braces getting in the way. He was prepping me to be a better lover for Jason Cooney.

One day, when we were in the hammock, I put my foot against his crotch and felt his dick stiffen. I kept it there. Soon after that, he suggested that I let him "prepare" me for the "real thing" with Jason Cooney. It hadn't even occurred to me there was something to prepare for—because my whole story was a ruse—so when Steve described how he could stretch me out a little, how he wasn't going to put the whole thing in, of course, just enough so that it would be less painful the first time, I was enticed.

We got naked from the waist down. He had built up muscles from playing water polo. His dick was big and veiny.

"This will be a good test," I said, encouraging him to get on top of me.

I was surprised by the weight of him. I could feel our pubic hair touching—his was rough—and the pressure, the reality, the muscularity of his penis trying to find its way in. For a few moments I felt a wonderful urgency, and I wanted him to get closer to where it was coming from.

"I don't think it's going to fit," he said. "You're really small."

I was both relieved and disappointed. Steve could see it on my face.

"Small is good," he said, smiling.

The urgency dissolved; his mood turned analytical as he suggested things I could do to prepare my small vagina for when it came time to actually do it with Jason Cooney, but I wasn't really paying attention.

I wanted to say to Steve: *You're my boyfriend, not him.*

THE NEXT DAY, while Steve was golfing with Grandpa, I was wandering around the property when I found my mother moving a pile of clothes from the main house to the cabin. When I asked her what was going on, she said she couldn't live in the house or eat with the family anymore—they were too awful.

"But you were just laughing with them."

"I was humoring them. They took all the good rooms," she said blankly.

"There are plenty of rooms," I said, walking toward the cabin.

"Not rooms with air. Chrissy, that fucking bitch, took the *one* room with air. She knows I can only sleep in that room." She grabbed my arm. "Aren't they all disgusting?"

I pulled my arm away.

"They're not *that* bad, Mom. You're overreacting."

She hadn't expected me to disagree with her. For a moment she looked hurt, but quickly snapped into fury. "I know you can't bear to be around me."

I wanted to say, *I can't bear to be around any of you.*

ONE WARM NIGHT after dinner, after everyone went to sleep, Chrissy, Franny, Steve, and I secretly went to the dock, took off our clothes, and dove into the black river.

Steve stood behind a chair while he undressed, and I laughed while I watched him from the water. I thought it was silly that he was trying to hide his body from me after everything we had done.

"What?" he said.

"I like to watch," I said in my Chauncey Gardiner voice.

He had no idea what I was talking about. He cupped his hand over his groin and cannonballed off the diving board.

In the water our voices sounded loud and breathy. We floated and looked at the bright stars and the lights from the bridge. Chrissy and I did an underwater somersault. Underwater we could feel the hum of an approaching ship.

Steve swam out toward the channel to catch its wake. As he moved away from me, farther into the dark, I was struck with nostalgia for the River. It was the end of the summer, and it almost hurt my chest.

Franny and I got out of the water to soap ourselves off on the diving board. We all used a bar of Ivory soap and the River as our shower.

"It's so calm tonight," Chrissy said, drying herself off and putting her white cotton nightgown back on.

Naked on the diving board, I made gyrating motions with my hips and goofy sounds while I lathered up my crotch.

Chrissy laughed and Franny said, "Eww!"

Steve was still in the water below. He looked up at me and whispered: *Grandpa.*

I jumped back in the River just as Grandpa stepped into the light.

"What's all this? Damn it!" he yelled. "Get your heads chopped to bits swimming out here at night. Who's that now in there? Get out!"

"Oh, Dad, it's just the kids, come on," Chrissy said.

"What was she doing there," he said, pointing to me, "with that . . . touching her . . . touching . . ."

I was treading water, naked still, waiting for him to go away so I could get out and get my towel.

"Touching her . . ." he stammered, and then gestured toward his own crotch. He stuttered when he said, "Her . . . belly!"

"Come on now, Dad."

Chrissy led him away, and we climbed out of the water and dried off as fast as we could.

But before they disappeared into the dark of the stone path, he suddenly turned around and started pointing at me and Franny like he was possessed. He was spitting again.

"You two . . . you touching your belly and making those sounds . . . get your heads chopped off, damn it all. Touching your belly like that . . . you, you . . ." He couldn't seem to get the last word out.

We tried to bypass him, hedging toward the house.

He finally spat: "You *whore*!"

Franny and I ran up the rest of the way and reached the front porch. The house was dark. My mother must have been wandering around because she had somehow heard the commotion and had caught up with us as we entered the house. Along the path I had, at first, been laughing with Franny, but when my mother asked me what was going on, I started to cry.

"What is it, honey?" she asked, scooping me up into her.

I whispered that Grandpa had called me a whore.

"Oh, *that* is it," she said, lunging toward him. "I'm going to make him apologize to you."

I leaped forward, quickly realizing what a mistake I had made. "No!" I yelled, trying to grab her back. "Mom, don't! I don't care, it was stupid, I don't even care anymore!"

"How dare you call my daughter a whore!" she yelled.

I pulled her toward the front door. Chrissy bear-hugged Grandpa to hold him back. My mother and I ran past the pool table, out the door, down the steep stairs, past the reindeer, across the front lawn and into the cabin, screen door slamming behind us.

Gaby, who had been sleeping in the cabin, lifted her head and said, "Too loud!"

We both got into bed with Gaby. My body was trembling. My mother's breath smelled foul. It clogged my throat. I turned my face to the wall so I wouldn't breathe it in.

"Don't be mad, Mom," Gaby said, fiddling with the buttons of my mother's shirt. "Gimme the tit, you bitch!" she said with a big smile, trying to make us laugh.

I snorted.

"That's an awful thing to say, sweetheart," my mother said, giving her the tit.

"Aaaand another summer for the anals," I said to the wall.

"It's pronounced ann-als, honey."

"Anals, ann-als, let's call the whole thing off."

"We are never coming here again," she said bitterly.

With the nipple secured between her teeth so she wouldn't lose it, Gaby said, "But ith my favwit place."

I turned my head to look at Gaby. "Of course we're coming back," I said.

I wanted to explain to Gaby that what happens at the River means nothing and everything, that we had been having these fights for eternity and then forgetting about them and then having them again. But I didn't have the words to explain why Grandpa calling me a whore was upsetting. I'd have to explain to her what a whore was. *A lady who does sex stuff for money*, I'd say. Why is that so bad anyway? And then I'd have to explain why it upset me that Mom got even more mad at Grandpa than I was. And why was that? I'd have to explain who Mom was.

Now

Last night's dinner was a success. We added a dash of THC tincture to our bourbon cocktails, gambling with our moods because being high around Mom can either spark curiosity and open conversation or send us into existential terror. Mom agreed to a drop as well.

The night had just the right amount of drunken conviviality, tears over lost time, and laughs over the absurdity of the past. At one point Cindy and Mom had their arms wrapped around each other and were tenderly kissing each other's cheeks and lips.

Cindy is now upstairs packing up to leave. We wouldn't expect her to stay more than a day. She's an unapologetic loner, and as much as I may have tried to push her in the past beyond the limits of what she can emotionally sustain, I'm moved that she's given this trip her all.

Gaby will head out tomorrow. Mom's flight is not for a few more days.

My mother and I now are sitting by the fire, present carcasses strewn around.

Lui enters the living room in a thong and tank top.

They wear thongs these days, the teens.

She shows off her body in a nonchalant way. It's an arresting sight.

Her brown doe eyes are accentuated with thick brows like Gaby's. Her curly chestnut hair is pulled back, exposing some bruising on her neck.

These teens, they shave everything until they are sleek and hairless. And they freely sport hickeys.

I sometimes "let" the teen girls see my naked body—my full bush, my hairy armpits, my granny panties, my saggy boobs, and my shamelessness about the whole thing. Depending on who is there, I might walk by Lui's open bedroom door in my underwear, no bra, and make a joke about the teen stench ("it smells like a medieval brothel in here"), maybe even wiggle my ass just to show them how comfortable I am with it.

I think of my nudity as a social service.

Lui plays the appropriately disinterested, sometimes-revolted teen; though, more recently, she has been asking me to show off my ass to her girlfriends. Apparently, they like my ass.

Right now I'm slightly on edge, worrying that my mother will ask about the bruises on Lui's neck. If my mother weren't here, I might say something like, "Why do the boys want to mark you like that?" But I won't dare call attention to her neck with Viva around.

I've asked about the hickeys before (but are those finger marks now?). I've tried to adopt the perfect tone: light curiosity, sarcastic disdain, and general not-caring-for-an-answer. I try to sound like the accepting mother with a dose of dark humor.

Oh, you have a hickey? Wow, the boys are such immature idiots.

She will usually hide her neck with a gesture of . . . what? Annoyance? Shame? No, not shame. This sex positivity is terrifyingly shameless. She'll say something like, "Shut the fuck up."

And then I will say something like, "Well, it's like a tattoo—if you don't want people mentioning it, don't get one."

But no, I would never subject Lui to Viva's thorough examination.

I know how Viva would have reacted to a hickey on my fifteen-year-old neck had I been lucky enough to get one and brave enough to display it. She would have dominated my body, taken my neck in her hands, and examined me with desperation, then thrown herself to the ground wailing like a Greek mother in mourning, exactly as I'd like to do when I see this hickey on Lui's neck.

Lui leans over the shabby chic couch and gives Viva a hug and a kiss. She's sweet with the grandparents.

My mother reaches her arm around Lui's bare lower back, glides her hand down to the crack of her ass, and snaps the elastic of Lui's thong.

"Oh, honey, how can you stand that thing up your ass like that?!" she shrieks as Lui walks away, swinging her hips.

"I know, ugh!" I say, laughing. "Me and Grandma love our nice big cotton undies."

I pat myself on the back for being on my mother's side.

"Well, good for you two hos," Lui deadpans as she marches proudly up the stairs, dismissing us.

"What did she call us?" Viva asks with genuine curiosity.

"Hos," I repeat with an air fellatio gesture.

My mother wails with laughter. "Ever since the anal cancer I can't have anything near my asshole. Oh, God! Remember how I had to use that awful dildo for the radiation?"

"What's a dildo?" Miko is asking, now cuddling up to me on the couch.

"A fake penis," my mother says.

As Nick brings Cindy's stuff to the car and everyone attends to their own business, Mom seems slightly stressed. A few days before any flight, she starts to freak out and obsess over things. There are generally a few trips to the post office to send things to herself that she doesn't want to fly back with.

"Marybeth is sending me a document to sign," she says. "And I have to get it notarized."

"Aha!" I say with an English accent. "I knew there would be no holiday trip completed without a visit to the notary!"

The only thing Mom likes more than visiting the post office is a visit to a notary.

"So you and Marybeth are in cahoots?" Gaby asks.

"Well, she agrees with me about the land," Mom says.

"Is Marybeth the scary sister?" Chris asks innocently.

"She's definitely the craziest one," I say and mouth the words *be-sides Mom*.

"She was married to Mom's ex-boyfriend Bob," Gaby tells Chris and Cindy.

"And now he's dead," Mom says to Chris. "Crashed his own plane into a field, killing himself and his young girlfriend."

"Jesus!" Cindy says. "What a story!"

Miko starts to chant "Fake penis, penis, penis!" as he marches around the living room. Lewis tries to crawl after him.

Rosy grabs Lewis and they writhe on the floor with abandon.

"Fako Penis! Fako Penis!" my mother chants even louder, banging her fist on the table.

Chris and Nick enter the room doing a *Riverdance* slapstick in sync with Mom's beat.

My mother leaps up and grabs Cindy's hands and leads her into a kind of ring-around-a-rosy skipping circle dance.

Cindy laughs wholeheartedly and joins the improvised penis song as

Lui runs back down to us in her thong and takes Gaby's hands, and Gaby takes mine, and now all the little kids are in the middle of our dancing ring, hysterical with joy.

I can't help but feel relief over having made it through the holiday so far, but the joy comes with a sense of loss, a mourning over our unfathomable souls and inscrutable minds.

Part 3

THE OUTER WORLD

1986–1989

Chapter 19

The Bump

t was in Mr. K's class, sophomore year, when I finally felt a warmth ooze between my legs for the first time. I was fifteen. At first I thought that maybe it was just from being so turned on by him.

Every day that year—after a morning in the basement of La-Guardia High School practicing the Stanislavsky method in a black leotard and tights with a group of other teenage actors, all of us chanting *ma na la tha va sa, may nay lay they vay say, mee nee lee thee vee see, mo no lo tho vo so,* praying for tears as we slowly waved goodbye to our loved ones on the deck of an imaginary ship as it set sail, and reciting "Out, damned spot! Out, I say!"—I then went upstairs, where I spent most of math class planning how I'd wait for my fellow students to leave before I locked the door, drew the shades, sauntered over to Mr. K, and sat on his lap. I imagined he would be in his swivel chair wearing his uniform—tight jeans and bedroom slippers—and before he could protest, I would gently thread my fingers through his messy dark hair and plant my lips over his lips, silencing his sarcasm, sticking my tongue gently into his mouth, and . . . well, the fantasy sort of dissolved after that.

The afternoon I felt the warmth, I excused myself from his class, locked myself in a bathroom stall, pulled down my jeans, and saw the bright red spot on my underwear. *Holy Lady Macbeth! Holy mother of Mary. Or was Mary the holy Mother of God?* I still didn't know, but I thanked the Ladies and Mothers for making this finally happen.

Yes, yes, yes.

When I got home that afternoon, while waiting for the Chelsea elevator, I checked out my reflection in the desk partition.

Dude, I said to myself, *all you have to do is get these fucking braces off.*

A wave of cramps arrived. I relished the pain as the elevator numbers lit up.

"I got my period," I said to my mother as I pushed open the front door and sidestepped between the bikes and the sharp wall.

"Oh, honey, congratulations!"

She set me up on the couch with a hot water bottle and called Ruth to tell her the news. I could hear Ruth celebrate through both the phone and the bathroom pipes. My mother brought me a cup of tea.

"Well, honey," she said, sitting next to me and holding my hand. "You could have a child now, can you believe it?"

"First I have to get these braces off," I said.

That very night my mother let me call the dentist on the fourth floor of the Chelsea who agreed to peel off all the metal as long as I promised to be fitted for a retainer.

I never did. Instead, I just stood in front of the bathroom mirror and lifted up my shirt and smiled at myself. I ran my tongue along my smooth, straight teeth.

My breasts seemed to defy gravity.

"Nice boobies!" Gaby said, reaching up, cupping one from underneath and gently jiggling it like she was checking for ripeness.

"Thanks, monkey," I said, proud she had noticed.

I was ready for something to happen.

EVERY AFTERNOON, after school, I followed roughly the same pattern: Rebi and I would meet out front where we smoked with the boys from the band the Mommyheads before making our way to Central Park.

We'd enter on Seventy-second Street, walk through Strawberry Fields, pay our respects to Lennon, and head over to the Meadow. As we wove our way around the little groups of bodies gathered together laughing and smoking, I'd see a couple making out. Two lucky bodies, graced by the gods of sex. As I passed them, I couldn't help but stare, practically diving into their entangled mouths, living for a couple of seconds in between their probing tongues connected by strings of saliva. Each time, I promised myself that tomorrow I'd lock Mr. K's door.

Rebi and I would lie on the grass, procrastinating.

But those pesky red numbers on the huge digital clock fixed to the face of a skyscraper never stopped moving. As they flicked forward, they churned up dread. The more dread, the less I wanted to move. I tried to conjure a vision of the apartment, and what Gaby might be doing, what my mother's mood might be. My body was uptown, their bodies on Twenty-third Street. Why was this an issue?

A few straggly old pot dealers slunk around and eventually squatted down beside us to try to sell us beer and/or a dime bag. We didn't drink after school, and we never bought weed from the

Meadow guys because everyone said it was oregano. Not to mention, I had vowed never to buy weed again because when we first started smoking it, I was chosen to be the one to try to buy a dime bag in the East Village. I chose a woman dealer I had seen before. I handed her a dollar and waited for my change.

"Honey, you owe me nine more bucks," she said. Jesus, how could I be so dumb?

"Right, right," I said. "I thought that was a ten."

She smirked at me. I didn't have nine more bucks, so I told her I'd be right back and prayed I'd never see her again.

On the way home from the Meadow, Rebi and I would pass the back patio of Tavern on the Green. If there was a cocktail party going on, we quickly tidied up our clothes, reapplied our lipstick, and slipped in through the hedges, whisking a flute of Champagne and some hors d'oeuvres from a floating tray, and chatting with a businessman for a few minutes before slipping back out and heading to the Columbus Circle subway entrance.

We continued to entertain ourselves by entering the subway cars separately; Rebi would play the single woman sitting alone, and I the deranged stranger who entered her car and suddenly sat on her lap, or toyed with her hair, agitating the other riders.

When I exited on Twenty-third Street, she stayed in the subway car. We no longer lived on the same block. The Squat had lost their lease, and the troupe had split up and scattered to different apartments. Now Rebi lived with Eva and Pisti on Seventh Street and Avenue A.

Exiting the E train, I'd walk past the Squat—now a construction zone and soon to be a Cineplex Odeon—and turn my head from the sight of the rubble as I made my way to the striped awning.

"Busy girl," Merle would say, passive aggressively, as I entered the lobby and passed her. While I waited for the gold elevator, I stared at the desk partition. Shizo and the Crunch had taped their flyers next to each other. I rummaged in my school bag and pulled out a pen. I drew a big X over the Crunch's flyer and scrawled: *you suck, love Shitz-zo.*

When I got into the apartment, my mother was on the couch reading the paper. She said, "This AIDS thing is really, really insane. I mean it's an epidemic. It's not just from blood. I don't think you should kiss anyone."

Nothing to worry about here, I thought, as I went into the kitchen to guzzle some milk and slip into another fantasy about kissing Mr. K.

I HAD BEEN kissed for real once (I didn't count Steve) by a sort of famous actor while I was on a five-week shoot in North Carolina. He was twenty and I was still fifteen. I had fallen for him while we hung out together in the makeup trailer. On my last day there he drove me back to the hotel, handed me a signed *Calvin and Hobbes* book as a parting gift, and kissed me. It was a real kiss, tender and slow, like on the soaps.

When I got home from the shoot, I relived the kiss over and over again from the top bunk in our shared bedroom, where the three of us spent countless hours with our secret desires, silver fishes slipping through our fingers.

My own dreams would unfurl just beyond my mother's swishing feet, just above her head, her frizzy hair like antennae trying to decode them. I wanted to keep them away from her, keep them unintelligible. I would wake up, exhausted, trying to adjust to the bland reality of our bedroom, where Gaby and my mother were entwined in their own dreamworlds just below me.

Gaby had her own desires, her own self-soothing methods that were similar to mine, it appeared, as she humped a pillow under the covers, right next to me.

My mother, on the other hand, had conjured her desire into something tangible: a bump on the bridge of her nose that she was currently fixated on.

IT'S HARD TO SAY EXACTLY when my mother began to wake us up in the night to examine the bump.

When she was researching Freud's nose obsession, she told me a story about Freud and some other man—a surgeon—who had decided that his patient's compulsive masturbation was due to a "nasogenital" connection that could be cured by a certain nose operation that the surgeon actually performed, and afterward she had chronic and profuse nosebleeds.

Back then, we ridiculed these men for operating on a woman's nose to cure sexual desire.

"My nosebleeds haven't cured my sexual desire," I said from the top bunk, knowing she would love this joke.

"Ha ha!" she said.

But sometime around when I started my period, she started waking us up in the night, worried.

It started with the eyes.

"Honey, I'm afraid my eyes are not closing all the way. They're going to dry out."

She called the plastic surgeon.

"Pitanguy says it happens sometimes in the beginning," she said, somewhat reassured, after she got off the phone.

But later, when we exited the lobby, pushing through the heavy glass doors with the wind sucking at her face, she winced and lamented: "Oh, the wind on my nose! I can't baaare it! The skin is too thin. I should never have gotten that nose job. Goddamn it!!"

I tried to ignore it at first, then reverted to the old tactic: "Remember? No more coulda, shoulda, woulda!"

Still, in the night, she would beg for me to come down from the top bunk.

"Tell me, honey, how big is the bump?"

"I can't see anything, Mom; just leave it alone—you're not going back to Brazil."

"There's no bump, Mom, God!" Gaby chimed in.

Then she'd ask me to check her eyes to see if the top and bottom lids were sealing shut.

I felt like I was standing on a bridge, somewhere in the fog, trying to decipher what dreadful thing was approaching.

"You shouldn't talk to all those women," I mumbled. She was writing an article about the horrors of plastic surgery, creating files, chronicling her own personal experience for *Vanity Fair.*

"I have to for the article," she said with a sigh of resignation.

Later, from my bunk, I could hear her in the bathroom early in the morning. "I'm going to have to go back to Brazil, girls . . . the skin is tight and shiny around it. See? They'll have to shave it off. Alex, will you come and have a look?"

I had to admit that, yes, there was, actually, a very small bump. Nothing very noticeable. A small bump on her once famous nose, the nose she said her father had hated, and so I had paid for her to go to Brazil to have it made smaller.

"It's barely noticeable," I said, hugging her quickly before getting back into bed.

After she examined it in the mirror, she would get back into her bed and soon call to me again, "Come here and cuddle with me, honey. I feel so sick and tired. I've got a migraine. Oh, God, would I love a Coke and a filet mignon."

I would pull myself from the fantasies and climb into bed with her, putting my head on her chest, and she would hold me close and jerk me in her arms every now and then to reiterate certain words.

"You are the sweetest (squeeze and jerk) most (squeeze and jerk) beautiful (squeeze and jerk) daughter," she cooed.

One night when we were curled together she started sniffing me all over. "You smell like tobacco," she said. "Have *you* been smoking?"

REBI AND I smoked every day. We smoked after school and we smoked at the clubs.

Dancing at the clubs was what we loved most.

We would meet in front of the Palladium. Eszter had brought us there first; as long as we were next to her and I hid my grid of braces (when I had them), the doorman, Haoui, always let us in. Haoui was a short white Brooklyn boy with a frizzy halo of hair who ran a cabaret in the Palladium where Madonna and the Beastie Boys performed.

With no metal on my teeth, we didn't need Eszter anymore.

Once inside we would move with the sea of bodies over square tiles lit from underneath. We never snorted anything or smoked anything other than tobacco—we just danced blissfully, for hours, sweaty, pelvic grinding strange men until it was time to eat at Florent with Eszter and Stephen, surrounded by drag queens, off-duty garbagemen, and other tired clubbers.

In bed, when my mother questioned me about my smell, I was soft toned—quick but not rushed. I said: "*Me?* God, no. It must be from all the other kids I hung out with after school."

A few days before this she had found a pack of Merits in my backpack. I didn't skip a beat when I said, "I'm holding them for a friend who has a really crazy mother."

I had mastered this type of lie. No extra explanations—they had ruined people, those additional sentences, those made-up details. The tone said it all. It meant: *You are the kind of mother who does not need to be lied to, I am the kind of daughter who doesn't need to hide anything.*

She rubbed her legs against mine and said, "Your legs are so rough! You didn't *shave* them did you?"

None of the mothers wanted us shaving. They said if we shaved, the hair would grow back thicker, but that didn't stop us because we suspected it was bullshit.

"That's weird. No . . . maybe it's from my jeans rubbing against the hair on my legs and making them feel stubbly?"

"Or your tights," she suggested.

She often came up with strange explanations for things, and I encouraged this because it let me off the hook. If I had secretly borrowed something of hers—her favorite Peruvian sweater—and then lost it at school—she would say "they" stole it. Someone who worked or lived in the Chelsea, maybe? Even though I was the demon thief, I would always let her believe it was "them," which I felt a little bad about, whoever "they" were.

I guess I'm the gaslighter now, I thought.

MY INTERNAL DIALOGUE grew more vicious than ever, and I had violent visions from the top bunk.

My mother flossed in bed, and the snapping sound made me want to hit her over the head with the cast-iron frying pan.

I imagined wrapping the floss around her neck and pulling it tighter and tighter until the veins popped in her temples.

The sound of her ankles constantly swishing together under the sheets incited images of butcher knives thrust into her chest, blood spurting upward, splattering the ceiling.

She ate in bed; the chewing sounds made me thrash around under the covers and imagine suffocating her with a pillow.

IT WAS TWO a.m., and Rebi and I were walking to the Chelsea, up Seventh Avenue from Fourteenth Street, after a night dancing at Nell's, our new club. We were sixteen, laughing, eating a slice. The empty streets felt like our living room. We approached the bright glow of the Chelsea forty-five minutes past curfew, but I had a plan.

When we pushed open the lobby doors, Bonnie stuck her orange bouffant out from behind the operator's partition.

"Have fun, girls?" she said with her breathy voice.

"Yeah, so much fun. Love you, Bonnie," I said as I hit the gold elevator button with the heel of my hand.

Rebi and I draped our arms around each other and looked at our reflection in the desk partition window. *Not bad*, I thought. We kept our long hair in a sort of half-up, half-down tousled do, and we never went without a certain light orange matte lipstick. Our uniform: tight Levi's, Doc Martens, tucked-in white T-shirt, and an oversize blazer.

"I guess I won the final battle," I said to Rebi, cupping my size D boobs and nudging her with my hip.

"Fuck you," she said.

When we exited the elevator, our laughter echoed in the halls. I imagined my eleven-year-old self jogging up and down the stairs with a newborn.

Now I'm the carefree reveler, I thought.

We tiptoed into the apartment, and I threw my mother's bathrobe over the digital clock next to her bed, so if she stirred, she wouldn't see the glowing red numbers telling her how late we were. It would make her question herself even when she was sure she knew what was going on.

Getting up the bunk ladder meant stepping on her bed, but the weight of my body depressing the mattress could wake her, so instead I contorted myself to get a foothold on the bunk ladder without touching her bed and launched myself up. Rebi followed my lead.

Gaby was gently snoring in the bottom bunk.

We sardined our too-tall selves, head to foot, on the single foam mattress and tried to fall asleep, but I got the giggles and gave them to Rebi. Sometimes it felt like life was just trying to fold our oversize bodies into too small spaces.

The next morning, as the sun rose, I heard my mother saying, "Officer, I don't know where she is! She was at one of those damn clubs! I want them all shut down . . ."

I jumped off the bunk cheerfully and called out: "I'm right in heeere!"

"Oh my God, you're *there*?!" she said, running back into the apartment to see for herself. The cops followed. "I thought you were missing!"

She looked at me, then back at the cops, then back to me. "I checked a little while ago but saw nothing in the bed. Officer, I must be going crazy. Early Alzheimer's."

"We were in bed this whole time." I glanced at Rebi for mental support. "It's weird—we even came home early."

"Officer, I'm sorry, my daughter was in the bed this *entire* time!"

The cops left and we went back to sleep, satisfied that she thought she was going crazy. But it was clear by the way she was moving around the apartment later that morning that something was building.

She came in and out of the bedroom with piles of stuff, moaning or mumbling to herself, asking me if I knew where something was. I answered as though I had never been asleep, my voice bright and alert. But when she walked away, I let my head fall back onto the pillow and tried to pretend to myself that the inevitable wasn't going to happen.

Finally, the inevitable, in the form of a shrill voice: "Girls, get out of bed! I can't take it anymore . . . I'm going to need some help around here!"

I jumped off the top bunk as though I had been electrocuted.

Gaby sat up in the lower bunk bed and rubbed her eyes. She was going on six with long, disheveled honey-colored hair. She didn't like to get up before noon.

"What's wrong with Mom?" she asked, sounding annoyed.

I rolled my eyes and made the crazy sign with my finger.

Gaby laughed.

Rebi unfolded her long limbs and jumped to my mother's bed and then to ground level.

"Viva, how can I help?" she patiently asked.

I tried to show her with my eyes that I was so sorry my mom was being a dickhead.

Gaby flipped on the TV, and after we were all done helping her clean, my mother finally burst.

"I just don't think it's appropriate for you two young girls to be out all night. It's dangerous!"

"Mom, it's no big deal. It's just a *club, God*! And we weren't out all night!"

"What club were you at again?"

"The Palladium!" I lied.

"I want to go to the Palladium," Gaby said, pulling her attention away from *Fraggle Rock*. "It's not fair!"

"I'm calling them right now. What's it called . . . the Passadium, what? Tell me. Panadium?" she asked, as she dialed 411 to get the number and called the club.

"This is Viva—*Viva*, Andy Warhol Superstar—do you know you are letting minors into your club?"

There was a pause while, I imagined, the person on the other end was trying to catch up.

"Well, I'm having you shut down!" she yelled and slammed the receiver down.

"Mom. You realize this is the same place you called *last year* to try to get me into Haoui's cabaret, right?" I wanted to add, *you fucking hypocrite*, but I didn't.

I rarely, if ever, told her how I really felt. There was no way to say the words—they were either too mean or I physically couldn't get them out.

ONE AFTERNOON, however, she threw a cast-iron frying pan across the kitchen, and I heard myself scream *fuck you* out loud.

It was shocking to hear the words in the world outside of my head.

As soon as I said them, I ran out into the hall, slamming the apartment door behind me. I had to make a quick decision.

Elevators? No time to wait.

Stairs? Yes, but up or down?

I could run down the stairs and jump into the mouth of an elevator along the way, but I worried that while I was inside the elevator, she would get into the other one and could be waiting for me in the lobby.

Or worse yet, we could both be dinged out at the same time, stepping into the lobby synchronized, and turning to face each other like rivals in a duel.

So I sprinted down to the sixth floor, shoved open the swinging door, and hid in a smaller tributary, listening for her next move.

She screamed my name down the stairwell—the swinging door slapped her voice back and forth from the hollow central hall to the padded acoustics of the tributary I was in.

I waited longer.

Soon I heard our own front door slamming shut.

I waited another moment longer, my hands shaking.

Someone laughed from the inside of the apartment behind my back.

I jogged down to the first floor—haunted by Nancy—and lurked for a moment in the enclosed stairwell that led to the lobby. There I listened for the chugging or the ding of an elevator. I wanted to be sure she had really given up and wasn't riding down to find me.

To be safe, I decided to bypass the lobby altogether; I shoved open the El Quijote doors at the bottom of the stairs, passed the Chiquita bathroom, made my way past the bar where Bonnie was nursing a cocktail, praying the manager wouldn't see me, and ran toward the front doors that led to the street.

Once I was outside, I had to squint my eyes against the brightness to see my hand—it was bleeding—it had gotten snagged on something when I stormed out.

I looked toward the lobby doors expecting her to emerge any moment, knees buckling with rage, screaming my name into the din of traffic.

I wanted to run to the Squat, but I remembered it was gone, so I slipped into the Healthy Chelsea food store and hid in an aisle, waiting for something to change.

It never did.

Now

I text Gaby: *Mom missed flight. Too "sick" to travel. Heading to Mom's favorite place besides notary and post office: Urgent Care.*

I take Mom and her croaking cough to the usual suburban Urgent Care location we always go to when she visits.

During the examination she tells the young doctor about her severe childhood ragweed allergy, her anal cancer ordeal, and how a few of her siblings are suing her—or she them, again it's hard to follow—over how the remaining Thousand Island property will be divvied up.

I sit on a chair in the examination room and space out, letting the doctor navigate this situation by himself. Good luck, young man.

I begin preparing for the no-departure-date marathon. The training is pretty simple. It's based on the hibernation habits of frogs. You basically hunker down inside yourself and slow your heartbeat and breath down so much that an inexperienced doctor would think you were dead if she were to take your vitals.

They put her on steroids and antibiotics, but they say she doesn't have pneumonia.

When we get back home, she goes up the stairs slowly, like the summit climb to Mount Everest, sans oxygen.

She heads into the kids' bathroom with the enema bag.

I can't stop myself from saying, "Mom, are you sure you want to do an enema? You *just* took Imodium!"

I hate myself for saying this aloud. It's a Sisyphean task to point out her junkie-like reliance on both stool softeners and hardeners. She's like addicts on the eternal chase for the right high, pepping up their lows with speed and dampening their highs with downers. Only for her it's Imodium and Metamucil.

She doesn't miss a beat. She says, "I had *anal cancer*, honey!! Everything is all fucked up from the radiation!"

I want to say that it was eight years ago, but I say "Sorry" instead.

I was in my late thirties when she called to say she had anal cancer. I felt a rush of excitement. I had been fantasizing about the Final Goodbye for years.

The Final Goodbye is our only hope for redemption. It must be the final one, though, not the second to last. If the person doesn't die after the forgiving ritual has transpired . . . well, then you are back where you started because you then have to live life with the person as though you've forgiven them.

Here's how it will go:

"I forgive you," I say.

"I forgive you too," she says.

I pause. "But I don't need forgiveness . . . *you* do."

"You're right, sweetie, I'm sorry," she says, then pauses. "But you did try to kill me."

Here is where imminent death is really important. Because only if they are about to be eternally silenced can you get in the last word.

I say, "I will always love you and you will live in my heart forever and I forgive *you* . . ." And that's when the death rattle must begin.

Once I am certain the death rattle has started, I quickly add: "And David Icke just made a public announcement that evil people are not

lizards, they are just plain evil; God says chemtrails are just condensation; 9/11 was not an inside job; and there is definitive proof we really did
land on the moon! Ciao! I love you!"

Cue Final Exhale in my arms. Done. The dead can't talk back.

As it turned out, though, the anal cancer was only stage 1, easily cur-
able. I was compelled to offer a couple of weeks of recalcitrant nursing,
tag teaming her care with Gaby and a friend.

I flew to Houston, Texas, where she was living in Aunt Chrissy's house,
close to MD Anderson Cancer Center.

Chrissy and John were traveling, so it was just the two of us in their
big well-appointed house where every surface was topped with framed
photographs of the family at the River, and where all the ailments of my
mother's entire life were vindicated and given a wide breadth in which
to resurface and air out.

It was the first time I lived with her again since I'd left home.

It was there that I made her aloe smoothies and skimmed the milky
water from the tops of pots of rice; there that I aimlessly roamed the
house examining the old photo collages of the aunts—long limbed in bikinis on the dock, pregnant and nursing on the boat, gathered around
Grandpa at the dining room table—and so many of us cousins—naked
under orange life preservers, ruddy cheeked and windswept; there that
she got fitted for the device we called "the dildo" that would protect the
walls of her vagina during radiation treatments; there that I held her
hand through the painful fitting while she made sounds that were exactly
like the sounds she made while giving birth to me; there that I filled the
prescription for the "lube" that would help her practice with "the dildo";
there that I discovered I was pregnant with the fetus I later miscarried.

Now my mother is asking for rice water.

Now my mother is asking for a Coke.

Now my mother is feigning shock and horror at the amount of food on her plate that I've delivered to her bedside, saying she could never, never, never in a million years eat all this food.

Now I go down to my kitchen and scrape some food off her plate and return it back to her.

Now my mother needs Metamucil.

Now my mother is saying that Miko's gecko tank is poisoning her.

Now the enema bag is swinging from the shower curtain rod in the kids' bathroom like the lightbulb over the skeleton mother in *Psycho*.

Hello, old friend, I say to it.

Chapter 20

The Little Girl Who Lives
Down the Lane

Rebi and I were spending most of our time in Alphabet City. Before Rebi moved there, we had been told the neighborhood was too dangerous to hang out in, but we soon discovered it was meant for us. The Ukrainian and Polish diners—Veselka, Leshko's, and Odessa—were cheap and delicious. We drank coffee milkshakes from the narrow newsstand on Avenue A while we strolled through Tompkins Square Park, people watching and smoking cigarettes. At night we were served at any bar, not only because we looked older than we were, but also because it was an unmonitored place and time. Not chaotic, just free.

The junkies who haunted the neighborhood and lined up around the empty lot next to her apartment building felt ominous but were ultimately harmless. The dealers who seemed to control the lives of these junkies lived in Rebi's building. They knew us by name. They looked out for us when we came home late at night.

When we finally unlocked the front door, Pisti would emerge from the living room, where he and Eva slept on a mattress on the floor. He would be wearing saggy white underwear and a white tank top, and he would look like he hadn't been sleeping. He would say, to make us laugh, "Time to make zee donuts," like Fred from the Dunkin' Donuts commercial, only with a Hungarian accent.

ON ONE OF those evenings, Rebi brought me to an East Village bar called 7B, to meet the bartender, Tim. He was costarring with Eszter and Rebi in Pisti's new play.

Rebi and Tim had a long scene together in which he played a life-size tree designed and constructed by Eva.

Tim gave her intense looks, Rebi said. She was intrigued by him but also disgusted because he seemed to be flirting with both her and Eszter, and she suspected he drank too much.

Behind the bar, Tim was aloof but gave us free drinks. He was a little overweight, and half of his left earlobe had been bitten off in a fight. He drove an old Valiant and had a dog that he claimed was a wolf. The "wolf" roamed the neighborhood alone and sat on the hood of the Valiant while Tim tended bar. Tim had a way of talking where he stretched out his sentences with a lot of hand gestures and pauses filled with *ah*s, trying to make simple things sound mysterious and more complicated than they needed to be.

I observed the next rehearsal. During breaks Rebi and I bantered with Tim. He was very confident, I noticed, for not being that attractive. After the bantering he stared at me from the other side of the room. I understood the attraction now that I was getting to know him, but it was also annoying the way he tried to make something deep out of what was happening when nothing was really happening. Or maybe something was. You couldn't totally be sure with him, and I guessed that was the attraction.

One night, after dress rehearsal at the Brooklyn Academy of Music, a bunch of us went back into Manhattan to drink and eat. Tim and I were sitting next to each other, legs lightly touching under the table. I realized that all my jokes and imitations that night were meant for him. He seemed to find me hilarious. I couldn't eat anything because my stomach was fluttering. I pressed my thigh a little more firmly against his while I laughed. Under the table Tim took my hand. My eyelids went heavy. Heat spread from the center of my chest to my armpits. I pressed my palm into his, and my heart began to thump wildly.

It was dark on Seventh Street when we left, and Tim pulled me back, away from the crowd, closer to him. Traffic was light. Next to us Tompkins Square Park was dimly lit by the streetlamps that still worked. I was much taller than Tim, and the difference in our sizes was awkward as we moved closer to each other. He whispered "*You*" and gave me one of his mysterious looks. He gently grabbed the front of my T-shirt and pulled me in.

We kissed.

For a few seconds I fell into his mouth and melted. This was the kiss I had dreamed about: knee weakening, center cleaving, dizzying.

Rebi!

I forced myself to pull away and quickly walked up to her. She hadn't seen us, nobody had. I was relieved. As we walked, I knew I couldn't tell her. My head was buzzing and my blood was lava.

TIM BEGAN WAITING for me in the lobbies of the fancy hotels where I auditioned for movies. To me, he always looked disheveled when he was displaced from his neighborhood, sitting in the hotel's plush, oversize armchair, but he would arrange himself confidently, owning the space around him, as though he had been living in the fancy lobby for a while.

When I exited the elevators, we would acknowledge each other's presence silently, my face involuntarily melting into a smile. As I approached, he remained in the chair, unmoving, drawing me closer with a stern look on his face, a mock reprimand. We walked through the lobbies as strangers, but once we exited into the spring air and interlaced our fingers, I dropped into an alternate universe. Somehow my insides were heavy, but my body was light. We held hands and floated. Floated and kissed. We floated into Central Park, always avoiding the Meadow.

We leaned against trees and made out under the new petals. We lay down on one of the grassy slopes next to the reservoir and embraced and kissed more. We made out sitting on rocks, while we walked, under construction sights, in church pews.

Sometimes we would drive in his car; the interior smelled just like his scalp. His fingers and mouth tasted like tobacco. My eyelids fluttered when his scruffy chin was against my neck, and my insides turned into inky pools. We would eat at diners, drink coffee, smoke, go to the movies, and make out in the dark.

I made fun of him to his face, mimicked his coded way of talking, and imitated other people for him, like my mother. He loved it when I made fun of him. "You . . . are so . . . *funny* . . . I . . . ah . . ." he would say, and I would say, "Yeah . . . I . . . am . . . so . . . ah . . . funny," and then we would kiss.

We kissed so much that I never felt very hungry. We sometimes walked and kissed all the way from Central Park to the Chelsea— where he would leave me on the corner and walk in the opposite direction so we wouldn't get caught.

When I separated from him and I was walking past the ghost of the Squat—a Cineplex Odeon—and heading toward the striped Chelsea awning, I felt the weight of the human body again, the tug of gravity, the sharp edges of the world.

One afternoon, after seeing *Dirty Dancing* in the theater, we kissed goodbye on the corner of Twenty-third Street and Eighth, and I told him I loved him. He held my face firmly in his hands and said, "You are so . . . you just . . . ah . . . I . . . ah . . . Bam! It's like . . . nothing and . . . Boom! Everything goes around . . . and then you . . . you . . . *you*!"

I thought I understood his language. The long pauses in between each word, I thought, meant something inarticulate. I imagined what he was describing was love because as cryptic as he was being, what he was saying felt right. I assumed he was scared of my age, and the rest I just pretended to understand. I could feel him watching me walk down the street, under the striped awning, into the lobby.

At the elevator I dug a pen out of my bag and scrawled *kiss my ass Shits-zo, love Crunch* on Shizo's flyer taped to the desk partition.

When I entered the apartment, Gaby was listening to the *Dirty Dancing* soundtrack. She was singing along to "I Had the Time of My Life." I joined her. We slow danced to "'Hungwy' Eyes," and she jumped into my arms and we rolled around on the floor together before we watched *Full House*.

I had the urge to tell her, to say "I'm in love," but I didn't.

WHEN TIM WAS DRUNK, it was especially hard to decode his monologues. He tried to tell me he was not *good*, or I was *too good*, or he'd done something unmentionable the night before—but I never tried to find out what he was doing on those late bartending nights. Maybe he turned into one of the junkie zombies—I didn't want to know.

We rarely ever went into his apartment. The one time I had been in there was when Rebi was apartment sitting for him, before we had started secretly seeing each other. Rebi pulled one of his many black hardcover journals from the bookshelves and showed me what she had already discovered. In the pages, taped in rows, were his thick, yellowed toenail clippings. At the time the journals had unnerved me, even repulsed me. I didn't want to think about the toenails and the drunkenness when I was with him. I knew, though, that I had to get closer to him in order to have actual sex.

For the first time we'd decided to meet at his apartment. I had to sneak into the front entrance of the building for fear that Rebi might see me from her window directly across the street. She still crushed on him and would describe to me the charged way he still looked at her. Yet I felt so certain about his love for me that I believed she was delusional, and I never even bothered to ask him about it.

His apartment door was open when I arrived. He was waiting for me in bed, dressed, napping, or at least pretending to. I was late and was supposed to be at Rebi's within the hour. I climbed under his musty covers. He said, teasingly, "Go to sleep," but I pulled him closer and kissed him.

It had been hard to visualize having sex with him; not just because I had never had sex with anyone, but because in my fantasies I couldn't quite place my body together with his shorter, wider build. No matter, though, I had planned to do it sooner or later with him. When we first met, he had been surprised when I told him I was a virgin.

"What about that teen . . . ah . . . heartthrob you . . ."

"Oh, him?" I said, waving my hand between our faces. "That was nothing—all we did was make out."

In bed, Tim cupped his hands over my breasts. I pulled him closer and tried to put my hand down his pants. I had never felt his dick in the flesh, and I was ready, but he embraced me firmly, this time more like a restraint, and again he told me to go to sleep.

"YOUR CHIN IS all rubbed raw, honey, what is this? Have you been kissing someone?"

My mother was holding my chin in her hand, pulling my face up close to hers, examining it. She had caught me in the ditzy mood I was always in when I returned from walking with Tim. I wriggled away, disgusted by the examination, but amazed she could know this, and also curious to see the evidence for myself in the bathroom mirror so that I could relive it. I was feeling so happy, so in love, that I let my guard down.

"He's older," I offered.

The moment I said it, I regretted it.

She was dipping raw fish in egg batter, then laying it down on a plate of whole wheat flour.

"How old?" she asked, sounding casual.

Fuck.

"Not that much."

Please, God, make her let it go, I begged.

She continued to batter fish. "Come on," she coaxed, "you can tell me."

"I don't know, like . . . thirty," I said. I shaved off a couple of years.

For about twenty minutes she was calm. She asked me a few sporadic questions while she fried the fish, about how I met him, where, et cetera. I tried to keep it vague.

"He's in the Squat play," I said.

Stupid detail! I yelled at myself.

She had just piled the fried fish on a plate when she abruptly turned around and blurted out with the shrill voice, "Oh my God, no! Have you had sex? Oh, God! You're sixteen . . . *sixteen*! He's too old! Give me his number right now. I want to talk to him."

Here we go, I thought.

I refused to give her his number. I tried my best to change the subject, to get out of her eyeline, but I knew she wouldn't let this go.

It went on like that for a couple of days. Whenever I came home, she inspected my face. "You've been kissing him, haven't you? Oh, your face is all rubbed raw from his stubble. God! That old man? I can't bear it! I want you to stop seeing him."

She started making phone calls. There was no stopping her trajectory.

She called Eva first. Eva was furious, disgusted with Tim, had no idea anything was going on between us, and gave my mother his number right away.

Rebi found out next, of course. I was mortified. I gathered the courage to face her, and when I saw her, I knew that lying to her for the past few months had created a deep rift in our friendship. Of course she felt betrayed, abandoned. It felt like I had come in and swept him away after she had discovered him. She didn't hide her pain from me; it was raw, her tears flowed, I was at a loss for words. I offered shallow comfort and contrition. Her despair and bursts of fury made me want to hide away. I had no excuse that sounded right. I only felt *I wanted this and I took it.*

My mother called Michel next. This was so embarrassing I wished to be living on another planet. Suddenly *he* was having a "meeting" with Tim. It was the first time Michel and Viva had collaborated on anything since they were first together.

When I questioned Tim about these "interviews," he said, "Your mother is . . . ah . . . she's very . . . she is a very intense woman . . . she knows . . . very *smart* . . . ah . . . yeah." He was even more cryptic about his meeting with Michel. Some kind of men's covenant.

My mother wasn't cryptic.

"He doesn't even tie his shoelaces! Oh, honey, he's just a slob, mumbling his way through life, filthy clothes . . . a total slob!" She took me into her arms. "I can't bear to think about him with you, rubbing your face raw with his dirty stubble . . . and those *filthy* fingernails. He can't even finish a sentence! My poor little baby," she continued, holding her arms out and making goo-goo sounds. "Come here and hug your poor mommy . . ."

I wanted to bury her alive.

I ARRANGED TO HAVE SEX with him. My mother and Gaby had left early for Mexico, and I had the apartment to myself for a night. I cleaned up and ordered Chinese food. While I waited for him to arrive, I started to watch a Jodie Foster movie called *The Little Girl Who Lives Down the Lane* while I fantasized about the uninterrupted night with Tim. Our first sleepover. I would do it. Once I saw his naked body, it would all make sense . . . he would take over, he would know what to do. We would have a leisurely breakfast and I would no longer be a virgin.

Tim was very late. When he finally arrived, we ate the Chinese food and cuddled under the covers while we watched the rest of the Jodie Foster movie. It was about a thirteen-year-old girl mysteriously living alone. A creepy older man, played by Martin Sheen, visits her and makes sexual suggestions. It turns out that she had killed her abusive mother by lacing her tea with cyanide. Martin Sheen comes out of the basement at the end of the movie and says he will only keep her secret if she has sex with him. She agrees but then also kills him with cyanide-laced tea.

Tim seemed distracted and distant as we kissed and watched the end of the movie together. Then he got up to leave. I was flustered. He said he had to go to a meeting with his acting partner, but it was two a.m.

"Is it that you feel like Martin Sheen?" I asked, sort of kidding.

He laughed and left.

I cried myself to sleep.

The next day I left for Mexico to meet my mother and Gaby at our friends Patsy and Joe's house in Zihuatanejo.

Chapter 21

Neptune

On my flight to Mexico, I daydreamed about what I might find when I arrived at Patsy and Joe's magical house.

On our trip there the year before, I had left early to go back to school, and my mother and Gaby had stayed on. When my mother had returned home very, very tan, I knew something was off. She had always been vehemently against tanning. In order for her to tan her white skin, there had to be some kind of powerful influence at work.

When she pulled a black *thong* out of her suitcase—it was made from two pieces of material twisted together (the twisty part was meant for her ass crack)—it had suddenly dawned on me: she had been seduced again.

Fred Beverly was a sun worshipper who did not believe in sunblock, so he had permanently dark and leathery skin. It suited him. People said he was a walking encyclopedia who moved money around, never went to bed before three a.m., reshaped people's lives, and traveled the world. He had a swoop of blond hair that fell over one eye and a uniform that the women around him adopted: a slim-fitting striped dress shirt unbuttoned at the chest, tucked into Levi's, and white canvas Vans.

Women apparently loved him, including a very famous gap-toothed model/actress, who sometimes joined him in Zihua. He never stayed at Patsy and Joe's house. Instead, he encamped at Tres Marias, a cheap hotel with cell-like bungalows on La Ropa, the beach down the road.

"Oh my God, you wore *that*?" I gasped. I couldn't hide my shock when she had dangled the strip of bathing suit in the air. We had always made fun of those thongs.

"Fred said these are the only kinds of bathing suits that look good," she had said, putting it on, and turning around so I could get a better look. She said Fred had wanted her to show off her ass. Fred had very specific ideas about the way things should look. The way women should look.

"I'm surprised you're not wearing the uniform," I said, sarcastically.

My mother caught a glimpse of her tan body in the mirror, and she was suddenly horrified.

"I can't believe I let him do this to me. Just look at my chest! I'm covered in cancer spots. I've ruined my skin."

I told her she looked good and not to worry about it.

"No," she moaned. "I'll get skin cancer now. How could I let him seduce me? I mean *Jane* can handle the sun—she's got that swarthy Italian skin. And she's young! But I should have known better."

"Who's Jane?" I had asked.

"Fred's *other* girlfriend," she said glumly. "He doesn't bring you-know-who to Zihua anymore. Jane comes with him instead. She *hates* the water—can you believe that? Anyway, she loves Gaby.

She wants to put her in a McGruff the Crime Dog video. A "Don't Do Drugs" thing—with Drew Barrymore."

"So now Fred and Jane are together?"

"Yes, but Jane is terrified of bodysurfing, Alex. Can you imagine being with Fred and not liking the water? Ha! Well, she finally left because she couldn't hack it anymore. All that waiting around at the beach. You should have seen me, though. I was in there all day. One wave after another. I took the really big ones too."

"I love Jane," Gaby had cut in.

I had a hard time imagining my mother putting up with all of Fred's late-night talking and partying.

"Well, I'd fall asleep in his room," she explained, "and then he'd go out later. Oh, it's *pathetic*—don't make me talk about it."

She had dropped the thong into the top drawer as though she couldn't decide if it might be useful again in the future, and nothing more was said about Fred. For the next year the thong lived in the top drawer next to the pantyhose egg until it was time to pack for Mexico again—this trip—and she pulled it out like it was a piece of dog shit and plopped it in her bag—"just in case."

As the city disappeared behind the clouds, I put my head against the cold plane window and felt Tim dissolve a bit too. My heart loosened its grip. I needed some time away from all of it. If Fred was in Zihua, I figured he would still be a seductive figure for my mother, and that meant she would be distracted.

WHEN I ARRIVED, I got into a cab and rolled down the windows, enjoying the familiar smell of the smoldering piles along the road to Zihua. Soon I was passing the coconut groves and heading to Patsy and Joe's house on Playa la Ropa.

Patsy first met my mother when she waited on her at Max's Kansas City. My mother knew Joe as an art dealer in NYC in the 60s.

Patsy brought Joe to Zihua around 1969 and together they built Casa Luna—a big open-air house under a giant palm roof, a palapa, surrounded by lush tropical gardens. They invited all their friends from New York to stay with them during the winters, and soon it was a happening place.

After Casa Luna was finished, they built a restaurant in town, Coconuts, where we would all gather in the evenings, under the white Christmas lights, surrounded by Joe's miniature dioramas in glass boxes set into nooks in the adobe walls, eating from Patsy's delicious menu, drinking margaritas and Coronas with lime.

They were unapologetic potheads and cigarette smokers, lifelong, high-functioning wake and bakers, and Gaby and I adored them.

Over the years Patsy and Joe had enclosed their bedroom and surrounded themselves with specific luxuries that they couldn't live without: air-conditioning, satellite TV (Joe was a cable news junkie), a king-size bed, cartons of Marlboro Reds, a large canister stuffed with fluffy weed, and cabinets filled with refills of their addictions—cans of Almond Roca, wheels of Parmesan cheese, and the arugula, endive, and romaine lettuce that we would bring them from the States packed in damp paper towels.

When I arrived, I found them lying, as usual, side by side on their king-size bed, a large ashtray in the space between their bodies, their backs propped up by a number of pillows, ankles crossed, under a large portrait that my mother had painted of them lying side by side on the same bed in the same position. The ashtray was full, and CNN was blasting on their satellite TV.

Patsy unrolled the extra virgin olive oil I had brought her from its beach towel wrapping and said, "Oh, goody!" with a cute, lightly high-pitched voice.

She was wearing her usual—a loose men's shirt over a sarong that fell open to expose perfectly tanned shapely legs. Her hair was always the same—bluntly cut at ear level and parted down the middle.

Her small, squinty eyes sparkled with delight as she pulled a hunk of Romano from the hollow foot of a flipper. "Be still my beating heart," she said as I held up a pink and gold can of Almond Roca and shook it, lifting my eyebrows.

"Let's eat some now!" Gaby said, jumping up and down on the bed, spilling the ashtray.

"Babes!" Joe called out to Patsy. "Don't let the kids eat all my chocolate."

He was partially kidding, but he also knew that after a couple days we would be acting like we had been living in Mexico for years, desperate, like them, for American luxuries. Joe was wearing his usual outfit too—shirtless with white pleated tennis shorts. He was a short and stocky Italian American from Chicago with blurry gray navy tattoos on his hairy arms and a gravelly voice.

"Kid, get over here!" he called to Gaby.

He and Gaby adored each other. They were like two old fogies. She slid up next to him and affectionately bit his "big Italian nose."

"God." My mother laughed. "I guess she's desperate for a father!"

"Or has penis envy," I said.

My mother and I had our private Freudian nose/sex jokes that nobody but us understood.

"Wowza!" Joe said to me as I stood up. "Where'd those boobs come from?!"

I did a catwalk for them, showing off my new body.

"Legs for days! Honey, a little bird told me you're recovering from a breakup?" Patsy gently asked.

Maybe it was the pot, but everything she said came out sounding sweet and sincere. I knew how Tim and I must have looked to the adults in my life, so I didn't mind her concern, but I wanted to change the subject.

"She woke up, he wasn't there, she hates that," Gaby said, doing it for me.

Patsy and I cracked up. Gaby was imitating Glenn Close in *Fatal Attraction*. Patsy and I had taken her to see it in New York. When the movie was over and we were walking out of the theater, a few people shook their heads at us in disdain and *tsk-tsk*ed as we passed them. It didn't even occur to us that she was too young for the movie. I told Patsy they were provincial idiots.

To distract from more Tim questions, I kept our *Fatal Attraction* act going. I grabbed Gaby and said, "I want a rabbit, Daddy!"

THE NEXT DAY I overheard my mother and Patsy gossiping in the kitchen.

"So I told him he would be sucking cock in Sing Sing if he dared to continue seeing her," she was saying, impressed with herself.

"Oh, Viva," Patsy gasped.

"I mean he didn't even have the decency to tie his shoelaces when he came to meet me!"

"So did you force her to come here to get her away from him?" Patsy asked.

I walked into the garden before I heard my mother's answer. I didn't want to hear anything more about how much she tried to intervene with Tim. What she told him made me sick. And even more sick the way she thought it was so funny. I vowed to never reveal to her that I cared about what she *thought*. I now understood, at least, that she had scared him away.

I wanted to let go of Tim—I could see our story had come to its end—and as I went through that process, I also wanted my mother out of the story, out of my bodily memory of all that had happened.

Luckily, the Brothers Beverly had just arrived in Zihua, and so my mother and I both had plenty of distraction.

IT WAS UNCLEAR, at first, if my mother and Fred had resumed their affair. She still flirted heavily with him, but he had arrived with Jane, who seemed to think she was his "official" girlfriend, even though he acted like he was single.

Complicating things further was the fact that my mother and Jane were the best of friends.

My mother, unsurprisingly, loved this kind of love affair drama, offering advice to Jane, giving Fred the eye, then ridiculing Fred when he walked away, then ridiculing Jane's Fred obsession when Jane walked away. As long as she was preoccupied with them, the drama was somewhat entertaining for me as well.

Fred's brother Ron had arrived with his girlfriend, Kathy, and her son, Mike. They had driven to Mexico in their VW van. Ron was everything Fred wasn't—tall, muscular, accommodating, and cheery. He was a gardener, maybe in his midforties. He looked like a blond Tarzan. I was intrigued.

My mother called Ron the Blond Bimbo.

Ron introduced us to his daily routine, and we followed it for the rest of the trip. Bodysurfing was the primary objective. In order to get to the bodysurfing beach, we had to be in his van no later than eleven a.m. He wanted us to enjoy ourselves, and we were indebted to his patience because getting my mother out of the house on time was difficult. Even though hours before the van was idling, she had been trying to cajole me and Gaby out of bed, worried we would "miss the nice cool morning air and the good light," we would still have to wait for her once it was time to head to the beach.

She packed enough stuff for what looked like a week's excursion into unpredictable weather patterns. Each time we were ready to pull out of the Casa Luna driveway, she would yell *Wait!* and run back into "the studio"—a separate building on the property—to get another sarong and maybe also a down vest in case she got chilled at sunset.

If Patsy and Joe had been driving us to the beach, there would have been a fight about this. They rarely went to the beach anymore, but the last time they did drive us, when my mother finally got into his Jeep, Joe said, "Jesus Christ, Vives!" He angrily pulled out of the driveway and out to the bumpy dirt road and added: "I mean how the fuck do you get anything done?!"

Joe, like Fred, had no patience for this kind of thing. Patsy tried to diffuse the tension with her stoned, lazy laugh.

"I don't know, Joe," my mother said, dryly. "I wonder the same thing about myself."

Ron, on the other hand, was always good-natured about how long it took my mother to do things.

On the way to the beach he would look at me while he was driving, his face framed by the rectangular glass of the rearview mirror. His smile unfolded along the right side of his face, charmingly crooked, making deep crevices in his cheeks. Each time he caught my eyes, I'd feel a pleasant little zap between my legs.

We would always stop for breakfast in town for banana licuados, papaya with lime, scrambled eggs with black beans, and cappuccinos, then return to the van, where Ron played reggae for the twenty-minute drive to Las Quatas—the perfect bodysurfing beach (according to the Brothers Beverly) and where we set up camp for the day.

Fred would arrive on his own. He never rode in the van, never waited for anyone. Bodysurfing was a serious business for the brothers.

Jane always came with us. She still hated the water, but she was trying to train herself to like it so Fred would commit to their relationship. She occupied herself with a black felt-tip pen and yellow legal pad, always working on the Neptune/concubine/lost seaweed girl script she was writing for a play we would all perform together at Casa Luna on my last night.

Gaby and I were in love with her. She had black shiny hair always cut in a soft layered bob, heart-shaped lips always glistening with freshly applied red lipstick, and she described herself as "an Italian girl with a good head of hair, a tiny waist, a flat chest, a round ass, and short legs with fat ankles." She cackled hysterically at all my jokes.

"Just *have* a baby," my mother told Jane, with a tone that made it seem like the simplest thing in the world. "It's just a ridiculous, bourgeois idea to *wait* for the perfect man. He doesn't *exist*, Jane. He doesn't *exist*. Just get pregnant with Fred's child and have the baby. The man never does anything *anyway*, so I don't know what you're waiting for."

Jane laughed and said that she wished she could be more like Viva, but she still couldn't help wanting a father for the baby she was so desperate to have. She was a big fan of my mother's mothering—in awe, she said, of her "fearlessness," the "independence" she allowed Gaby, and her apparent "indifference to men."

While Jane waited for the father of her future baby, she focused all her maternal energy on Gaby. She made up rhymes and fairy tales and knew hundreds of songs by heart that she could call up at any moment. And she wrote plays for us. Writing the plays was a great excuse—she joked about this—to *not* have to go in the water. Instead, she could spend all day at the beach, plodding away at the script, she said, "only getting my fat ankles wet."

I was addicted to the waves. From under a palapa I'd watch the Brothers Beverly bodysurf for a while, assessing the day's swell. I could see their blond heads bobbing in the water as they waited for the next wave to crest. When a good wave arrived, their heads would lurch forward ahead of the wave, the wave would grab them, suspending them for a moment in the clear water just before it broke, and then they would disappear in the white foam until they slid up onto the shore

When the waves were huge, Fred and Ron would give rides on their backs to those of us who were willing. You could choose either brother.

I had a certain kind of love for Fred, but I did not find him attractive. I was amused by his little shirtless body in the glare of the noonday sun, curled on his side on a tiny Tres Marias towel, empty white canvas sneakers placed neatly beside it, taking notes with a black felt-tip pen on a yellow legal pad, chain smoking Parliament Lights. I found his lectures entertaining for a while, then dreadfully repetitive and boring, especially after he had had a few drinks, and he tried to tell me some theory about my soon to be revealed genius, even once drawing an unintelligible diagram on a cocktail napkin that was meant to decode, or encode, my movement forward in life parallel to the growth of my breasts with some cosmology sprinkled in.

During dinner one night I imitated Fred's cosmic tit talk for the group; I hunched over a napkin with a felt-tip pen and mumbled with a gruff voice, "OK, you've got this and that . . ." here, I gestured to Patsy's tits and then made some squiggly lines on the napkin, "and when you get here, you'll know you're there . . ." I manically drew some black circles . . . "and there is where you see . . . that is this." Even Fred had to laugh.

I chose to ride Fred's back only when it seemed like I was riding Ron's too often. Ron and I would enter the water separately and wait, sometimes treading water, sometimes digging our feet into the thick sand beneath, turning our heads to the horizon, squinting from the sun, looking out past the fifty-foot jagged rock formations that rose from underwater, searching for a good wave.

We would float over the crests of the unwanted waves in silence, the giant rocks in the distance witnessing how we rarely spoke at all.

Sometimes we would glance back to the shore where we could see, but not hear, our friends and family sitting under the palapas.

When the right wave began to roll in, we would make eye contact; then Ron's rough hands would be on my hips, guiding me behind him, our bodies skimming against each other. I would hold his waist as we pushed off, synchronized, until the wave caught us both and we were momentarily both suspended inside the crest of the wave before it broke. As it propelled us forward, I would wrap my arms around his slippery muscles. My breasts and my belly hovered just above his body, a saltwater boundary between us, our skin sometimes making contact. As the wave broke, we were shuttled out to the front of the wave and my body would glide against the back of his, my hands sliding up to his hairy chest, where I could feel his heart pounding and the foam churning underneath us. As the wave slowed and brought us to shore, his calloused hands would always reach up from underneath and slide, first over my waist, and then even more slowly over my ass, as we were finally delivered to the wet sand. Before we separated, we would pause against each other for one extra moment before the water pulled away and left us exposed.

Ron gave everyone rides—Kathy, Mike, Gaby, my mother, and whoever else might be on the beach with us that day—but I never wondered if he might glide his hands in the same way over Kathy's or my mother's body. Kathy rarely entered the water. She sunbathed and when the sun began to dip below the horizon, she would start getting irritable. We could see her from the surf, see her shading her eyes with her hand, looking out at us in the water and starting to pack up the stuff. That was how we knew it was time to get out and head home.

Once we were all packed back in the van, pruned, starving, and thrillingly exhausted, Ron would crank the reggae again and look at me from the rearview mirror with his rubbery smile.

Tim felt like the light layer of salt left on my skin.

AT SOME POINT I felt Mike's hands grabbing at me underwater. I was repulsed by the twelve-year-old version of copping a feel. His stunning confidence coupled with his squat little body disgusted me. I was offended that he even attempted to get my attention this way. I did my best to avoid him in the water.

When a good wave approached, I tried to get as close to Ron as I could while Mike tried to grab on to me, wanting a ride on my back or, ridiculously, wanting to give me a ride on *his* back. I was at least two feet taller than him. I wanted to laugh in his face, but I still felt a little sorry for him, so I did let him ride my back now and then. Underwater he would sometimes try to slide his little hands down the length of my body, and I had to stop myself from turning around and whacking him on the head.

The adults thought of him as an innocent little boy, and one person even suggested that when the mosquitoes were keeping him awake in his hammock bed, he should climb into bed with me, across from my mother and Gaby in the studio, under the mosquito net.

When Mike got into my bed, I would never kick him out or tell him to keep to himself; instead, I had violent fantasies, similar to what I felt toward my mother from the bunk bed at home. I wanted to squash his self-satisfied face between my hands and say, *Do you even realize I'm in love with your stepfather, you stupid little fuck?*

I WAS A concubine in Neptune's cave, my arms draped around his neck. We were still, waiting for the seaweed "curtains" to open. Joe had designed the set. Gold, red, green, and blue metallic strips rippled in the warm ocean breeze. I could feel Neptune's heart thumping under his bare chest, thumping against my own chest. I wore a silk floor-length negligee that dropped low at my cleavage.

It was performance night for Jane's play.

In the morning I had to return to eleventh grade, but Gaby and my mother would stay on for a couple more weeks.

Neptune grunted softly—soft enough that the audience couldn't hear—and looked down at me. His large hand brushed over my ass. I swooned.

Gaby was on the other side of the metallic strips of curtain— onstage—the lost seaweed girl, dancing to haunting violin music in the underworld.

Our mother was downstage, the fortune teller/witch, wearing a gold turban on her head, standing in a shimmery silver tube of material, conjuring a spell.

Neptune and his concubine emerged from the cave.

The set was lit with tall white candles and clusters of birds-of-paradise.

Jane narrated from a bamboo throne, wearing a tight satin kimono, the script in her lap. She said, "The End," and the audience—the neighbors—stood up and clapped and cheered.

Later, after we celebrated, I shirked away when Mike tried to put his arm around me as we walked through the garden to the studio. My mother and Gaby were already in bed.

I had planned to wait for twenty minutes before I got up.

"Where are you going?" Mike immediately asked. I wanted to say, *None of your fucking business, little boy,* but instead I mumbled, "I need some water."

Most of the lights were out in the main house, but from where I stood in the garden I could see some light shining through the slats of the bamboo wall around Ron and Kathy's loft bedroom. I walked very slowly between the palm leaves and looked at the stars, waiting until Ron appeared.

Earlier, I had imagined we might say something to each other first—talk about the moon or the play—but he only grunted and took me into his arms without hesitation. At first it was strange to feel lips other than Tim's, but his hands felt wonderfully heavy on my ass and the kiss was as I had imagined—long and slow. While it was happening I fantasized about us sinking down onto the dewy lawn, hidden from the house, his weird goat body over mine, his hairy, calloused hands cupping my breasts . . . *Would this be an appropriate place to lose my virginity? Would we be caught? By*

Kathy? What if Joe came out—would I want to be caught by Joe while losing my virginity? Would it be a good losing-my-virginity story? Worse, what if Mike caught us . . . worst of all, my mother . . .

I broke the kiss and walked back to the studio. I got back into bed with Mike and lay very, very still.

ON THE WAY to the airport my mother rattled off some errands she wanted me to do: "Tell Stanley he has got to get that vent cleaned this month. And, honey, don't forget to deposit that check. I left some cash in the top drawer. Oh—and can you call . . ."

I was relieved she was there and talking because I knew Ron and I had nothing to say to each other—we had only ever exchanged a few words/grunts—and her voice took up the awkward space. I caught his eyes in the rearview mirror; the focused reality of them pulled me away from where I preferred to be—in the fantasy of *what if*. What if I had taken this further . . . what if we pursued this when he returned to New York.

I looked at his creased face. On dry land I felt much less attracted to him. His shirtlessness, his age, his goofy smile, his cheesy reggae. Desire was like a drug, I guessed, coursing through your system, turning on everything, making you loopy, desperate, urgent . . . until it just dissolved without warning, emptied you out, left you at best with indifference, at worst with revulsion.

Desire possesses and then abandons you, I thought.

Now

Don't crack, bitch.

How long has it been?

This is a deep freeze.

I've just been to the drugstore for Metamucil (the old container having been lost in the piles of stuff around her bed), eye lube, and shoe
inserts.

I've got rice on the stove for her rice water.

Oh, she'd love some flan too.

Maybe a steak as well and a baked potato?

Not too much on the plate, though.

I've been here before.

Now I'm standing in my upstairs hall putting the clean towels in the
linen closet.

This fucking linen closet.

I've always wanted a linen closet. Seemed like a sign of success. Now
that I have one, though, I can't get it to look like the linen closets I had
fantasized about. Other people in this family put things on top of the
sheets and towels—things like toilet paper and hard objects I can't figure
out because it's too dark in there.

What's this? A plastic pump? Hair clippers?

Everything in my linen closet ends up in messy piles.

Successful people use labels, I guess.

My mother is in Miko's room, talking on the phone.

Lui's bedroom door is ajar, and she is sitting on the edge of her bed making out with a boy.

I'm still for a moment, tempted to gape at them, in awe, the same reaction to people making out that I had when I was a teenager.

How free she must feel to kiss like that, in her own house, with the door open.

To be so bold as to leave the door open! No interest in hiding it from me.

Is this healthy?

I have the urge to close her door to hide the scene from my mother's eyes. But what would that be telling Lui?

I walk away.

When we were recently in family therapy, I sat still on the therapist's couch and listened while Lui described how she sometimes feels at home: filled with anxiety, unable to relax, ill at ease, no privacy, subjugated by our unpredictable moods, eager to get away from us. According to her, we are loose in some respects, highly demanding in others.

Mm-hmm, I said, straight-faced.

Inside, I was dying a slow death. This is an inventive form of torture—hearing your child's version of their childhood. I had to assess how much to say. I said not much.

I fear that trying to not be like Viva has made me remote.

"I feel like when you think I'm exaggerating, like when you don't really believe me—that's when you say 'Mm-hmm,' like that," she said.

While the therapist nodded encouragingly, I hoped for a large meteor to wipe us out.

I set boundaries, didn't I? I never talked about my sex life in front of her, I never asked her advice on where to live, what to do . . . while remaining kooky, loose, and spontaneous, hadn't I?

Then the therapist asked Lui if she had a clear grasp on what my childhood was like. While we waited for Lui to answer I felt confused about what he was getting at. Did he want Lui to know that I'd had a strict upbringing? Or was it more laissez-faire? What was my childhood like? You tell me, I wanted to demand. Was he suggesting that Lui's childhood was easier than mine? Or was he suggesting I am a fucked-up mother?

Now, as I walk into my own bedroom and close the door, I find myself thinking: *She can't relax?* Making out on the bed with the door open feels pretty relaxed to me.

No privacy? Close the door.

Does she not appreciate how much freedom she has?

Attachment parenting, check. Nursing on demand, check. Free to be, check. Intelligently progressive, check. Sensibly scientific, check.

Now I sound like Viva.

The night when my mother paced the streets of Tivoli, back when I was in college, ranting like the town crier, I could hear her voice while I was hiding in a closet.

"Daughters!" she orated. "If you have a daughter first, keep on trying to have a son. The girls will end up hating you. And you will never understand what you could have done to deserve it. Pray for a son. A son will fight your battles for you. All I've ever done is help people. My whole life. That's all I've ever done. And what do I get for that? My daughters hate me. What have I done to deserve this? Did the Holocaust victims ask to be gassed? Did the Rwandan children ask to be hacked to death? Just like Delphine Serige said, twenty years ago—did Jesus Christ deserve to be crucified?"

I had vowed to never say words like this to my own child, but I can't escape the thoughts. Raising a daughter does feel like a crucifixion.

Shut up, Viva.

I didn't say any of that in the therapist's office. I just sat on the couch and looked into Lui's eyes.

I hear my mother's voice calling out from Miko's bedroom.

"Honey, I think I'm dying."

Chapter 22

"Run for Your Life"

D ude, I've got to stop saying *dude*," I complained to Rebi.
We were in her Seventh Street apartment with Anna, our
new friend, listening to the Beatles. We were in early sixties–
inspired outfits, getting ready to go out and do our "thing." All
year the three of us had been performing around the city as The
Gore Triplets. Anna was a petite blonde, so we choreographed a
dance in height order, teased our hair, wore vintage shift dresses,
set ourselves up in front of the outdoor seating of crowded Soho
restaurants, an empty hat on the sidewalk, and sort of sang/lip-
synched to a boom box playing the song "Maybe I Know" by Les-
ley Gore. Strangely, we were a hit; even the Mommyheads invited
us to open for them at a couple of their own gigs.

"I just think it's sick," Rebi was saying about the Beatles song
"Run for Your Life." "Is he threatening to kill her?"

"They all have weird ideas about women. Let's go," I said.

Things were OK between Rebi and me mostly because Tim was
now going out with Eszter, and so we bonded over our shock at this
strange and unholy turn of events.

We fluffed our bouffants, grabbed the boom box, and walked to Soho.

That night we made more than a hundred dollars. We split it, left the boom box behind the desk in the Chelsea, and went to the Limelight to dance.

When I returned home the next day, the front door was wide open, the bikes were thrown into the outer hall, and all my mother's suitcases were lying open on the living room floor: sarongs, bikinis, tubes of sunblock, flippers, towels, paints, and piles of sand on the rug.

Gaby was in Sydney's apartment, and my mother was lying in bed, moaning, not making any sense. It was hard to tell whether she was happy or depressed.

"Oh, honey," she said, "thank you for cleaning up."

I had left the apartment spotless before I left the day before.

"What's wrong?" I asked.

"I shouldn't have come back . . . but I missed you too much."

"What do you mean?"

"I don't know . . ." She rolled over and moaned. "Oh! I can't take it!"

I had never seen her quite like this. The winter sun was low in the sky, weakly finding its way in through our greasy windows.

"Did something bad happen?" I asked.

"No, no . . . you should have seen the big waves I was taking. Huge! Just huge! After you left, Ron really got me going on them. Oh, we had such a great time." She paused and took a breath. "Kathy never goes to the beach. She just shops in town. It's so pathetic."

Something wasn't right. She had liked Kathy before I left. I started to put stuff away. She kept flopping on the bed with a strange, pained, yet euphoric expression on her face. She was beginning to really annoy me.

"Maybe I should have stayed," she lamented.

"Oh my God, Mom! Why are you acting so weird?"

"I think I'm in love."

OK, so it was good news—she was in love with some cool Mexican dude, she would be preoccupied, easy to handle. We would have a second home in Mexico. Things were falling into place.

"Yeah? Really? With whom?"

"I can't say."

"Come on, are you kidding? All this and you 'can't say'? You know you *have* to tell me, right? A Mexican dude, right?"

"No."

Oh, duh, it must have been Fred again and she couldn't say because of Jane.

"Fred, right?"

"He's practically married."

"Oh my God—did Fred marry Jane?"

"Not Fred, the man I'm in love with already lives with someone."

She was driving me insane. I tried to think of all the married guys we had run into in Mexico.

"It's Ron," she finally said.

I paused.

So it's unrequited love, I thought. *This is weird and unlike her, but it's unrequited love and that's why she's in turmoil.*

"Did you tell him you loved him?" I asked, trying to get to the point—that he didn't feel the same way, obviously.

She didn't answer.

I was feeling very impatient and very agitated. I was thinking about what a fool she was to have fallen for those gorilla grunts of his and those dumb-ass deep gazes.

I mean, at her age she should know better. Even I have gotten over him, and we actually had something together. She must be an idiot to have fallen for the same guy as I did—I mean, for one thing he's out of her league and for another . . .

"He's in love with me too . . ." she finally said, and then with a shrill, alarming tone she added: "Oh! I miss him so much . . ."

No. I must have heard her wrong. Or she just doesn't know what's going on—she is just imagining that he loves her . . .

"Did you have sex?" I asked. This would make it clear to her that they didn't have anything because of course he would not have had sex with *her*. I was so convinced she would say no that I almost didn't listen to the answer.

"Well, you know, *Kathy* was around, but we would be in his van and at the beach and Kathy *hates* the water. Then she went to Mexico City to *shop* for a few days—all she ever wants to do is shop—and . . ."

I don't know what my face looked like at that point—I tried my best to hold it in one neutral position. "And you had actual sex in those places? In the van, et cetera?"

"And at the beach . . . and honey, you can't *believe* the waves I took. Waves as big as you were taking, I really got into it, you know? Oooh, I miss him so much! What should I do?"

"Just lie down for a while and get some rest . . . I have to get something at the deli."

I ran down the seven flights and tucked in my chin as I marched through the lobby, praying Merle or Stanley wouldn't stop me.

OK, OK, OK, I said to myself as I stepped onto the sidewalk. Suddenly I was the Unmarried Woman about to puke in the gutter.

You want her? Go ahead, dude, be my guest.

I walked slowly toward Seventh Avenue, speaking to Ron in my head.

What is the deal here, dude? You are a sick fucking asshole, that I know.

I shifted the order of things in my head. I felt sorry for her, really, to be stuck with such a complete dick. I knew it wasn't her fault, how could she have known? But also, *She must never know!*

He's sick, I thought.

Oh, this would kill her.

Or it would kill me if she knew.

He has no shame, I thought. *He's some kind of sex addict, maybe.*

Any last remnants of attraction I may have had for him completely evaporated. He was fucking my mother, so he was dead to me.

I rearranged the order in my head so efficiently that by the time the gold elevator *ding*ed me back out onto the seventh floor, I had already figured out that I could play it out to my benefit. This calculation quickly dissolved the weight of the betrayal.

I had not seen my mother in love since I was a little kid—*I curse the day Bill and Bob and Fred and Ron started walking the earth*—but I knew exactly what to do.

"You girls should go to the park, it's such a beautiful day," my mother suggested. She was acting coquettish—it was her way of pretending to keep a secret. Normally she would have *never* suggested we go to the park without her. And we were not idiots. Gaby and I smirked at each other.

She had just returned from a food-shopping spree with three huge flower bouquets, mangoes, cherries, bread, cheese, and a hunk of pork she intended to roast. When we questioned her more about the feast, she said, conspiratorially, "Look, Ron thinks you girls don't know—let's just humor him, OK? You'd better go before he gets here."

"Gross, Mom," Gaby said.

It was unfolding exactly as I had intended. Gaby and I could wash our hands of all the guilt we used to feel leaving my mother alone in the apartment. In fact, we began to encourage her to prolong her afternoon trysts for as long as she wanted to, making sure we relayed the right amount of subtle irritation at being displaced. That would weigh down her side of the guilt scale in a tangible way.

Soon every weekend was ours alone. When we left the apartment, she would always say, "It's terrible how you girls have to leave the house . . . I should just get rid of him . . . it's just awful . . ." and I would feign reluctant dismissal: "Oh no, no, don't worry about us, you enjoy yourself."

It was too good to be true. We simply could not get in trouble no matter how long we were gone.

The downside was that we had to listen to her on the phone describing exactly what went on when we were out on our walkabouts. Apparently it was "*incredible* sex" and they fucked and ate all day. They dined picnic style on the living room floor, surrounded by the flowers. She would prepare these feasts for hours before he arrived, roasting lamb, mashing sweet potatoes and rutabagas, making mango salad and peach pies.

When Gaby and I got home, the remnants of the feasts would be spread around the house, and my mother would be wearing her blue velour robe, her hair tousled, her face flushed, her mood easy. She would greet us at the door smelling like sex, and say, "Girls, I'm sorry you had to stay out all day . . . oh, I wish I made enough money to buy us a big house so you could have your own rooms. Come here and kiss me . . . oh, nah-nah, goo-goo . . ."

The messes would throw me into silent rages but cleaning up was better than having to live with the remnants of their trysts. So rather than wait for her to do it, I would wash the dishes, tidy up the living room, pick the scraps of mango skins off the kitchen floor, shove things into drawers with a violence I found satisfying, while excoriating her in my head.

ONE NIGHT I climbed into my top bunk and nestled under my blue down quilt only to smell sex all over it. It was concentrated right at the top edge where my face was.

I pushed the comforter down to the end of the bed and used the sheet for warmth.

When it happened again the next week my heart raced. I dug in to find words: "Um . . . my blanket seems dirty?" I managed to say.

I was scared to ruin her mood, or to make her get up, or to have to listen to her apologize, or to obsess over the affair.

"Sorry, honey, I had your blanket on the floor today . . . want mine?"

I wanted to rip the blanket to shreds.

Instead, I lay there, unmoving, with shallow breath, and said: "No thanks."

MY MOTHER SPOKE to Kathy almost every day on the phone. Kathy complained to her about Ron. He had an ex-girlfriend who lived near his gardening business in New Jersey, and Kathy was unhappy that he spent time with her.

"Just ignore it," my mother advised her.

Meanwhile, my mother would hang up and get obsessed with the ex-girlfriend herself.

I knew this wasn't going to end well.

"She's just so typically Dutch," my mother complained one night after having had dinner with Ron and Kathy. She still continued to hang out with both of them at their apartment. "The whole apartment smells like Clorox, she's constantly wiping down tables, obsessed . . . it's unbearable . . . *such* a ridiculous neat freak. *Constantly* wiping down surfaces. But then *she* smells funny, you know?"

She had always been obsessed with searching out the source of weird smells. Lately the smell of shit, in particular, had been cropping up.

"Pew!—I smell something *shitty* in here," she would often say, or "I couldn't stand talking to him anymore, his breath smelled like *shit*."

Some white guru had recently moved in down the hall from us, and he told my mother that when you are enlightened, you can smell other people's impurities. She took this to heart, became friends with him, even hosted a night of chanting in our apartment, and then Gaby started doing a possessed dance around the house while chanting in Sanskrit: "Satguru Jyota Se Jyota Jagao!"

My mother continued about Kathy: "Yeah, there is something about her smell . . . *sour.* Even though she tries to keep everything so clean, she smells. The way she obsesses over what Ron has been doing all day—God! Yuck! I don't know how he can stand her. Well, let's admit it—he's not that smart. Fred got the brains in that family, right, Alex?"

"Right. He's an idiot—that's why you're sleeping with him."

"Right! Ha! He's a blond bimbo."

If she caught me in the right mood, I was still willing to gossip with her; I would talk about our friends and their horrible eating habits. But most of the time I lived in my own head and just repeated the last words she had just said to make it seem like I was participating—*unbearable, disgusting, I don't know how you took it for so long, pathetic.*

ONE SPRING NIGHT my mother and Gaby had returned home from a dinner at Ron and Kathy's. Gaby burst in the door and announced: "Mom got a huge injection in her nose! It was disgusting!"

Apparently, after dinner they had all smoked a joint, and when my mother started talking about the bump on her nose, a doctor who was there suggested injecting it with cortisone. He said he could do it right away. He had his medical bag and a syringe with cortisone.

Ron had said they were all crazy.

Kathy thought it was a great idea.

Gaby was playing cards with Mike, and she said that when she walked into the dining room, the doctor was sticking a "huge long" needle into the side of Mom's nose—right into "the bump."

"It was so painful," my mother said.

"It was really gwoss," Gaby added. "I tried to stop her."

My mother went to the mirror and examined her face. "He says it will shrink the bump."

Great, I thought. *Anything to get her to shut up about that fucking nose.*

"And now Mike is coming to Iowa," Gaby said, rolling her eyes and making the crazy signal with her finger.

Over the summer she would be playing Kevin Costner's daughter in a movie about a baseball field in Iowa. I would be paid to be her on-set guardian for a week before I returned to New York to be in a movie that Eszter was starring in.

"You're kidding, right?" I asked Gaby.

"It was Mom's idea," she said, shrugging.

"Mom?" I said, demanding an explanation.

"He has nothing to do over the summer and Kathy is a nightmare."

It was exasperating how difficult my mother made things. I suspected she wanted Mike there so she could be even more entangled with Ron and Kathy. But she would never be able to hack it with Mike, I knew this. She would get fed up with him, he would grate on her nerves, she would freak out at him about something, and Gaby and I would have to deal with the aftershocks.

Now

Carole, Nick's mother, is here. She was a high school English teacher for the majority of her life, but when she and Nick's father divorced, about fifteen years ago, she became a therapist. We get along great, but I worry that the fact that she lives just blocks away from us rattles my mother.

There is something on the radio about the #MeToo movement and to make her laugh, I snort and say, "Every guy I ever fooled around with I could #MeToo now."

I've forgotten that my mother is right in the other room. She hears this, of course, and immediately comes into the kitchen, excited.

"Oh, God, Alex! Carole! Me too! *Ha ha!* I mean Ron Beverly gave me anal cancer!"

"Well," I say, "that's not exactly a MeToo moment."

"What is it then? I didn't ask for warts!"

Lui is now in the kitchen making herself some ramen.

"Don't listen to her, Grandma. My mom is always on the boy's side," she says. "He could be like a serial killer rapist, and she would say, 'I feel bad for him, maybe the girl made a mistake?'"

My mother is cracking up with Carole.

"I regret the sex I had with every single man I've ever been with, Lui. Total waste of time," my mother says.

"And you never get lonely, Viva?" Carole asks.

"Are you kidding? Of course I do! I'm horribly lonely, just waiting to die. But I'd rather die than sleep with another man. Eww! Oh, disgusting, I can't even think about it. I don't know how you do it, Carole. You still date men, right? Well, you're younger than me, aren't you?"

"Not by much," Carole says.

"It's the Italian skin, I guess," my mother says, examining Carole's face. "Or you've had work done . . ."

"Not much," Carole laughs.

"Val has the good skin too. Does she still have an eating disorder?"

Carole laughs this off too, plays dumb. She never lets my mother get to her. Twenty years ago when we were all here in Philadelphia for Thanksgiving, Val, Nick's older sister, took my mother to a Chinese restaurant for lunch on Thanksgiving day, and my mother decided she was food obsessed and has never stopped talking about it since then.

"But, Grandma, if you never had sex, you wouldn't have had Gaby and Alex," Lui says.

"Ha, right, Lui. You are so smart. But Alex and Gaby hate me now, so what good did it do me? I guess your kids don't hate you, Carole."

"I wouldn't be too sure, Viva," Carole winks.

"Well, I'm never having kids," Lui says.

"Good for you, honey," my mother says. "You only have kids so someday there will be someone to take care of you when you are old."

Kill me now, I think.

"I didn't know you had cancer, Grandma," Lui says.

"You didn't know?! Well, you were too young to remember. Your mother left you in New York so you wouldn't miss school."

She is examining a black-and-white photograph on the mantel. She picks it up to look closer. My friend Layla and I are standing outside on my old stoop, naked and pregnant, framed by ivy on the West Village town house.

"I would just take your mother and Gaby out of school whenever they wanted," she says, still looking at the picture. "In fact, I moved to wherever they wanted to move! I did everything they wanted, and now look, they hate me for it. Great shot. Who is this? This pregnant woman next to you?"

Stay in hibernation, it's not spring yet, stay down, down, down.

"It's Layla," I say.

"Oh, the lesbian."

She puts the photo on the coffee table, not back in its place, and heads to the bookshelf. I know she's trying to see if any of the books are hers. Books we may have "stolen" from the storage space. The two books that she wrote, specifically. They are out of print now. Her own eye on the spine of *Superstar* catches her attention, and she pulls it from the shelf to examine it, trying to decide if it was once her own copy.

"I've got to go lie down," she says, taking it with her. "I'm exhausted."

"Let me make you some tea," Carole says.

"Carole, don't get up! You've been working since six a.m.," I interject, wanting to add *while you've been lying in bed, Mom.* "I'll make you both tea."

Chapter 23

The Dent

I was apartment sitting for one of the actors in a movie I had just been in. He was married to a woman who'd starred in one of my favorite childhood TV shows.

Though my apartment-sitting duties were minimal, I had already killed a plant and almost starved a cat. When I finally let myself in to try to save the situation, I persuaded Rebi to join me.

We spent hours snooping around the apartment until we found gold: her address book. She had every teenage heartthrob's number. Sitting on her bed, we tried calling Rob Lowe. He picked up.

"Hello?" he said.

"Hiiii, babe," I said.

He paused. "Who's this?"

"Ha. I miss you. You never came to the party."

"I didn't? Remind me: What party?"

"You're in a funny mood tonight, hot stuff."

We went down the list of numbers doing this routine with whoever would pick up the phone. We copied Rob Lowe's and C. Thomas

Howell's numbers down, took the dead plant to throw in a trash can a few blocks away, and left some extra cat food out.

A few days later I had to return the keys to her husband, a flirtatious Texan whom I found both sleazy and sexy.

When I arrived, he was alone in the apartment wearing a cowboy hat and tight jeans. We chatted about the shoot. I was wondering if he was going to mention the missing plant, but he kissed me instead. While we kissed, I decided I was going to get it over with. He was surprised when I told him I was a virgin because during the shoot I had talked about going out with Tim, whom he knew from the acting world, so at some point he assumed I was more experienced and probably that I had a thing for older men, which I guess I did . . . or, I joked to him, they had a thing for me.

As though he was preparing an altar, he laid a white towel on his wife's bed for me.

To capture the proof, I thought.

When he pulled down his jeans, I was much more shocked about what I saw than he had been about my virginity.

Dude, no way, I thought.

He must have seen the look on my face because he said, "I've been told it's bigger than average."

Oh, Jesus, I thought.

He couldn't find a condom, so I said, "I guess we should wait, then."

And he said, "It's OK, I know what to do."

I'm so sure, I thought. We hadn't even started, and I was already rolling my eyes.

"I've never had sex with a virgin," he said.

"You haven't?" I said.

"No." He laughed. "You seem so surprised. I mean it's not like I do this all the time."

I hadn't said it because I was surprised—it was just a conversational filler because I was so nervous about the limb trying to enter me. I needed him to shut up so I could concentrate. Or maybe his stupid banter was a good distraction.

He tried to be gentle. He seemed to enjoy it.

I, on the other hand, felt almost nothing but uncomfortable fullness. I had assumed the penis would give me the life-changing orgasm I had . . . what? Dreamed about? Read about? And I assumed the penis orgasm would be a different feeling from what I had already been giving myself.

When I was on my own, I was used to lying facedown, but now I was on my back, staying perfectly still to avoid pain from the giant dick. There was something familiar about this stillness, similar to the mute and catatonic state I sometimes kept myself in, on the top bunk, to avoid committing matricide.

Afterward he offered to do it again, as though he would be performing an act of service.

I wanted to say, *No way in hell, dude, is that thing ever getting near me again*, but instead I said, "No thanks," and I got ready to leave.

I saw him checking the towel. Yes, there was a spot of blood. *There it is—the lost virginity. Out, damned spot! Out, I say!* I thought, smiling to myself.

"What are you smiling about," he said flirtatiously, trying to embrace me.

"Nothing," I said, limply hugging him back. "That was nice."

"Did you cum?"

I wanted to say, *Dude. No. But don't worry, I can keep doing it on my own, like I've been doing since I was four,* but instead I said, "It was . . . intense."

"I'll call you later?"

"Yeah," I said heading to the door. I let him kiss me before I left.

He did try to call me, many times. When I saw him in person, he tried to question me about why I wanted nothing to do with him.

Isn't it obvious? I wanted to say. *You captured my lost virginity on a towel on your wife's bed. I'm seventeen and you're . . . whatever—thirtysomething—and I used to masturbate while pretending to be your wife.*

Instead, I never spoke to him again.

GABY WAS SIX going on sixteen when she returned from Iowa. She had fallen in love with Ray Liotta and was convinced he loved her back.

As I had predicted, things went terribly with Mike. Mom said he allegedly set something on fire on the set and sent him home. She had decided he was a sociopath, and of course this caused strife between my mother and Kathy, and then between Ron and my mother because Ron was not exactly in line with my mother's theories about Mike.

By the time my mother returned from Iowa, Kathy was not speaking to her and Ron was keeping his distance.

Around the same time, Anthony sent Gaby a picture of himself— a glossy black-and-white professional headshot signed *Your Father*, which the three of us made fun of.

"He is such a narcissist," my mother cackled, staring at the picture.

"What's that?" Gaby asked.

"Someone who only thinks about themselves. But you look just like him," my mother said. She was convinced he wanted a piece of Gaby's potential fame once the movie came out.

Gaby had to spend a certain number of court-ordered weekends with him. I was personally willing to consider that he just wanted to get to know her, and I had sometimes been acting as the liaison, negotiating with him over the phone about pickup times, and so on. I joined Gaby for her first sleepover at his apartment, which was awkward, but we managed it together.

After one weekend visit, Gaby had returned home with a white American Eskimo puppy. Mom thought it was psychotic that Anthony would buy a dog without asking us first, but luckily she let it slide after Gaby begged her not to give it back and promised Mom her own firstborn if she didn't follow through and take care of it herself.

We named it Tupi after one of the abandoned Topanga Canyon dogs. Tupi immediately took a shit on the Oriental rug and when my mother screamed "Goddamn it!" Gaby and I startled, cleaned it, grabbed an egg, and took the dog out for a walk.

When we got to the stairwell, I gestured toward the key shoot, Gaby unlatched the little door, dropped the egg in, and we jogged down the rest of the way.

It was the winter of 1989, my last semester of high school. Gaby and Mom were in Chicago for another movie shoot, *Uncle Buck*, and I had the apartment to myself.

I ran into Vincent Gallo, the artist I used to lust after when I was a kid at the Squat. He could hardly believe it was me, he said, I had grown up so much. He asked if he could pick me up at the Chelsea to hang out.

He called up to the apartment from the lobby. I took the gold elevator down and found him standing in front of the desk partition in his uniform—brown pants, white T-shirt, brown jacket, and brown fedora. He was dressed like an Italian Mafia man from the sixties. He had longish black hair, but his eyes were a ferocious blue—penetrating, almost icy. I thought he was stunning.

"What's this about?" he said, pointing to a press clipping that Stanley had laminated and taped to the glass partition. It was an article about famous people living in the Chelsea featuring my mother and Gaby, but my mother's face was partially covered with black marker.

"Oh, that?" I said laughing, pulling him away. "My mother did it. She doesn't want to be used for publicity unless Stanley reduces our rent."

On the street we fell into performing pranks for pedestrians, as though we had been working together for years. He would almost always dictate the conceit of the prank: he was usually some sort of forlorn man with a limp, and I played his daffy new bride.

This could work, I thought. *Yes, he's older, but I'm legal, and we get along.*

It was the first of several outings. In the beginning of these afternoons, I felt certain we would return to his apartment and fool around. But he never made a move. Meanwhile, he raved about my beauty and humor while I continued to lust after him.

Most often I would meet him in his apartment on Elizabeth Street, where, out front, he had written his name into the cement. Inside I spent endless hours pretending to be interested in his art when all I wanted to do was kiss and have sex. I was dying to try it again with someone I was actually into. I felt confident I could use the penis correctly the next time I had the chance. To get the chance, I figured I had to do my penance: examine the grapes and vines he etched into pieces of metal, pretend to be wowed by his rare guitar collection, his vintage motorcycle suits, his sound system, and his love of Chet Baker.

I pretended I wasn't disturbed by his closet—pristine rows of ironed and military-like folded brown pants, white T-shirts, white underwear, and brown jackets.

I read the beginning of a script he was writing, an autobiographical thing that took place in Buffalo, where he had grown up.

Still, he wouldn't even kiss me. He said I had a dirty mind, and sex would "sully" our relationship.

"I can't have sex with anyone I love," he insisted.

Bullshit, I thought.

He was interested in my acting career and seemed flabbergasted that I had lost the part in *Dangerous Liaisons* to Uma Thurman. The movie had already come out and there was a scene where Uma was topless. He asked me to show him my breasts so he could compare them to Uma's. I showed them to him enthusiastically—hoping they would peak his interest in sex. When he saw them, he said, "Oh my God—are you kidding me? They gave the part to *her*? Those are perfect."

Yet still nothing.

"College is for idiots," he would say. "Do you want to be a dough-ball or a star? College is designed to hold people like you back. You should keep acting. *Make money.* Uma is *nothing* compared to you."

I became paranoid at times, convinced he was gaslighting me. One night after he had encouraged me to hang out, I walked to his apartment and buzzed and buzzed, staring at his name—*Vincent*

Gallo—in the square of concrete, but he never answered. Finally, I walked back home, openly sobbing along Seventh Avenue.

It felt like a breathless ghost was trailing me, lonely.

When I unlocked the apartment door, the phone was ringing, alarmingly. It was my mother.

"I don't know what to do," she said with a heavy, dark voice.

I assumed she was going to say something about Ron, about how he was pussy whipped by Kathy, that he had officially broken up with her, or that she wanted to call Kathy to tell her everything.

Before she left for Chicago, Ron had stopped coming around. I'm sure he was terrified my mother was going to rat him out. I didn't blame him because Kathy and my mother were now enemies, and all my mother wanted to do was talk about how fucked up Mike was.

See what you got yourself into, I wanted to say to him. She was my revenge.

"Do about what?" I asked, dreading the conversation, blood draining from my veins, eyelids going droopy, guts heavy.

"It's absolutely freezing in Chicago. Arctic. I can't take the cold on my nose. When the wind blows, the skin on my face tightens up . . . Oh, Alex, I can't take it. It pulls where the scars are. Oh, why did I ever go to Brazil?" She was almost crying.

So it's the wind on the nose, again.

"The cold actually hurts your face?" I asked, trying to sound sincerely concerned.

"It's totally *unbearable.*"

"On your nose?"

"On all the scars. My eyes—they won't close all the way—they never have, you know, since Brazil—but with this Chicago wind it's just unbearable. And now there is a small dent on my nose, and in the cold it just throbs and throbs . . ."

"Can you wrap a scarf around it?"

"I think I may have to come home . . ."

"But what about Gaby?"

"I know, I know. I feel terrible about it. But Joe's niece—who lives here—said she could be Gaby's guardian."

After I hung up, Bonnie rang and said I had missed a call from Vincent. When I called him back, he said he had been at the neighbor's the whole time and why hadn't I called out his name from the sidewalk?

"I hadn't thought of it," I said, feigning indifference. I was worried he was gaslighting me.

THREE DAYS LATER my mother returned to the apartment.

During the next month, while Gaby was in Chicago, she researched the effects of cortisone. She pulled apart her filing cabinet and pored through the Plastic Surgery file that held all the interviews and medical journals she used for her *Vanity Fair* article. She read that, in large quantities, cortisone can atrophy the skin.

She kept trying to call Kathy to give her the third degree about the doctor at the dinner party, but Kathy kept hanging up on her.

In the dawn hours I inspected the nose for her. I would feel her by my bedside in her flannel nightgown, as I had when she obsessed over the bump, her hand heavy on my shoulder.

"Honey, I'm sorry . . , I'm sorry to wake you up . . . Allie? Would you just come under the light and really take a good look? Honey, can you just look and tell me the truth. Do you see the dent?"

I could see a tiny little shiny dent on the side of the bridge of her nose.

"It's minuscule," I said. "Try to get some sleep."

I was like a manatee that sleeps with half its brain awake and one eye open, but if she saw the eye open, she would start in as though we were in midconversation.

ONE NIGHT SHE SAT UP in bed and said: "It was Kathy."

I stilled myself and kept my breathing sleep steady, but she continued.

"She sabotaged me. The dent is from that *fucking injection* that quack gave me. Dr. Salatin. The cortisone. I can't believe I fell for it. She must have orchestrated the entire night! That dinner! She must have known about Ron and me back then. Well, that's it. It will completely atrophy. I've lost my nose. Oh, that cunt, that *miiiiiiiserable cunt*!!"

When she said "miserable," she dropped her voice to a lower pitch, almost a growl, teasing out the first syllable. "Honey, my nose is destroyed!"

I got into bed with her and held her quivering body. It felt frail. She was so vulnerable, so distraught that I softened.

"Mom, no, no, it's not true. Your nose will be fine. Kathy doesn't know anything. I swear—it's *nothing*."

Once the sun rose, she began to plan some kind of attack. "Kathy just hung up on me. I'm going to Dr. Salatin's office today. I'm going to sue that cocksucker. They both set me up. The skin has atrophied. Ron won't get on the phone. He's totally pussy whipped. What did I ever see in him? Am I crazy? Tell me the truth," she said, staring straight at me. "I'm crazy, aren't I?"

Yeah, you might be, I thought, but I didn't answer.

I TOLD VINCENT nothing of my mother in her nightgown in the apartment. I told him nothing of the bump and then the dent. I just waited for him to have sex with me, but he wouldn't, and then I would walk home with the lonely ghost trailing me, trailing me and siphoning my breath from the hollow dent in my own chest, siphoning the breath to bring it back to my mother.

"Come here, honey," my mother said, taking my face in her hands. "You seem so unhappy . . ."

"I'm not."

"You're not?"

"No."

What is she trying to get at?

"Why?"

"You just seem a little depressed."

She was inspecting my face, and I was trying to keep my expression neutral.

"Well, I'm not," I said.

"I should have let you stay with Tim."

"What?" *Jesus, where the hell is she going with this?*

"You were so happy with him."

"What are you talking about?"

I tried to turn away, but she pulled me toward her.

"I scared him away . . . and then you . . . you slept with someone you weren't in love with . . . some *married* man . . ."

Jesus Fucking Christ.

She looked desperate. I actually felt bad for her. I was about to reassure her that I was not depressed over my wasted virginity—just to shut her up—when she said: "You left your journal open on your desk. I feel so terrible . . . You were so happy when you were with Tim . . . You said it yourself . . . I should have let you sleep with him . . ."

Should have LET me? I repeated to myself with disgust.

I tried to maintain a stoic expression while I imagined spitting in her face, holding her by the neck, and smearing her spit-covered face with the dog shit on the rug. I quickly tried to remember everything I had written in that journal. My stomach slid into my feet, and my feet sank through the floor when I imagined her reading all the secrets I had stupidly written down. I broke away from her, mumbling something, and left the apartment. I didn't wait for the elevator. As I walked down the stairs, I realized the horror of it all was that she wasn't exactly wrong.

She called Ron at work and told him about Kathy sabotaging her. He was fed up.

When she hung up, she cried, "How could I have let that idiot seduce me? I can't stand the sound of his voice. Oh, he makes me sick!"

For weeks she trailed around in her nightgown, moaning and looking at her nose in the mirror.

"That bimbo!" she called out to the apartment. "What was I thinking? Kicking you girls out of your own home . . . spending all our money on those elaborate lunches . . . I'll never touch a man again. Oh, to think! I was totally brainwashed by the sex. Ron came on to you, didn't he? It's OK, you can tell me. Will you come in here and cuddle with me? Oh, honey, I'm so depressed. Alex, think twice before you ever get involved with any man—they're all bastards, selfish fucking cocksuckers. And on top of it all my nose is destroyed."

Every lament ended with: *and on top of it all, my nose is destroyed.*

There were a few moments when I was tempted to use her weakened state as ammunition. I imagined while she was so frail, that it would be easy to rail into her, to list all her faults, to say, "I told you so. And by the way, he did seduce me first and I figured out much faster than you that he is a sick fucking moron from hell."

But there she was, in that flannel nightgown, reaching out to me, her voice softened, saying, "I'm sorry. I'm depressed. That fucking cunt Kathy sabotaged me. I don't know what to do. I can't go on. I'd rather be dead. Honey, I'm sorry to do this to you, but I'm having a nervous breakdown."

A nervous breakdown. She had said this before, and it meant nothing.

I examined the dent, the almost invisible hollowed-out pit at the bridge of her nose.

I tried to reason with her, to list all the great things in her life, most obviously Gaby and me.

I tried being firm—*Just stop it,* I once said, as though I was angry. This tactic actually propped her up for a couple of hours.

"You're right, honey," she said. "Don't worry about me. You can go out. I promise, I won't kill myself. I was just saying that. Go out and have some fun."

So I did.

Before I walked to Vincent's apartment, I checked my reflection in the partition. I could see that my front tooth had distinctly popped forward from the premature braces removal. I pushed on it with my index finger. I thought about what Vincent said: a snaggletooth adds character to a beautiful face.

She had a dent and I had a snaggletooth.

I don't know what changed, maybe I tried to kiss him that night, or maybe it was because I had turned eighteen, but finally he said, "You want me to fuck you? Yeah?" I said yes and while he did it, he said, "I'm fucking you, this is what you want? I'm fucking you . . . I'm fucking . . ."

I looked up at him while he narrated the sex, then I turned my head to look into his closet—which was right up against his bed, the door ajar—and when I saw his folded brown and white clothes, I almost laughed out loud. I had never been talked dirty to before and it sounded so silly.

Is this turning him on? I wondered.

He seemed angry.

And here I am on my back again.

When it was over, he turned to his side.

I reached around to cuddle him, thinking he might soften if we actually kissed.

We had still never kissed.

"What? You want to kiss now . . . OK . . . Fine, let's kiss."

I couldn't figure out what this game was. He kissed me passionately; it was the kiss I had been dragging myself over there for; the kiss that made me pretend to like his cold metal etchings; the kiss that compelled me to listen to his endless guitar playing and sigh over his boring songs; the kiss that drove me to admire his closet of stupid vintage motorcycle suits while secretly rolling my eyes; the kiss that broke the spell.

I walked home and decided I'd never speak to him again.

WHEN THE ELEVATOR *ding*ed open, I prepared myself for what might be waiting for me on the other side of 710. Before I got to the door, Sydney came rushing out with her finger to her lips, shushing me. She gestured for me to listen at the stairwell. We could hear the Crunch practicing inside their apartment on the sixth floor. We tiptoed down the stairs and opened the breaker box on the sixth floor landing and pulled a few switches until the hall lights went out and all went silent.

"Motherfucker!" we heard a man yell and an apartment door creak open as we ran upstairs, cracking up.

When I got to the apartment, my mother was still in her flannel nightgown, aimlessly standing in the middle of the living room, looking at me seriously.

"Maybe you should just commit me. Honey, I'm sorry, but I'd rather be dead. I can't go on. I think I need to be committed."

I stared at her, trying to decide if I should really take her seriously, hoping for a sign that would guide me. A sign from the dent, if the dent could speak.

I'll pack her a little bag, Jerome can hail a cab, she'll stay in the psych ward for a couple of weeks until she feels better. Gaby and I will obviously be fine without her. On the other hand, they might not let her out of the psych ward and she'll end up a mess— drooling on her hospital gown, playing with her own poop, and Gaby will be motherless . . .

I took the phone. The mouthpiece smelled of foul breath. I called a wealthy friend of hers.

"We need help," I heard myself telling him. "We need a psychiatrist."

Saying it aloud made me sick.

I handed her the phone.

The people on the other end talked about the side effects of lithium and Prozac. They talked about Epstein-Barr.

She talked to her old friend Abbie Hoffman—he was depressed too. He told my mother that his life after the sixties revolution had been meaningless. They talked about how they had never received any compensation for all their work, and what was the point of doing anything?

"You're invisible when you're old," she said.

He told her how the drugs had helped. At least he can get out of bed now, he said.

So she began to take lithium.

Every time the little pill went into her mouth, I coaxed it into her bloodstream, hoping for peace, hoping for quiet, hoping to be released.

THERE WAS A LITTLE PROGRESS. A little room to breathe.

She was different. She was easier.

She didn't completely like herself on the lithium. She asked me what I thought. What did I know? When she asked me if she seemed . . . spaced out, dazed . . . I stupidly said: "*Yeah, maybe, a little.*"

A few weeks after she started taking the lithium, Gaby returned from the *Uncle Buck* shoot. We got in bed together and watched *Charles in Charge*. We were singing the opening theme song like we always had, with exaggerated enthusiasm: "Charles in charge of my life, of my days . . ."; there was a pause toward the end of the song there—and that was our favorite part—"I want . . . (pause) . . . I want . . . (pause) . . ." and that was when we started manically singing until we were in a frenzy for the last line: "Charles in charge of . . . *me!*"

My mother walked in and announced: "Abbie is dead. He committed suicide."

We looked up at her sympathetically, unsure of what it all meant.

"I guess lithium doesn't work after all," she said. "Should I just stop taking it?"

We didn't know. We didn't want her to die. Sure, I had fantasized about suffocating her, but actual death? Suicide? No, no, no.

She had always said, "I'm just going to kill myself," but we hadn't taken her seriously. It was a refrain.

This felt real.

Was she saying that lithium caused Abbie's suicide?

"You better get off it," we said.

What did we know?

ONE AFTERNOON THERE was a knock on the door. I opened it to find Jerome holding out a package.

"Thanks," I said.

"No problem," he said and walked away. He sounded sarcastic.

My mother began to unwrap the package with the violent, haphazard, jerky motions she opened all packages with, like she had just gone blind. She pulled out a long narrow object wrapped in pink tissue paper. Gaby and I pulled ourselves away from the TV set to watch.

She unrolled the tissue paper and held up a large, flesh-colored rubber thing.

"Is that a penis?" Gaby asked, seriously confused.

"Dude!" I said, laughing. "It's a dildo!"

"What's a dildo?" Gaby asked.

"A fake penis," I said.

"Let me have it!" Gaby screamed, jumping up to grab it.

My mother had been quiet so far. She quickly opened the letter taped to the dildo. There was a long pause.

"It's from Kathy," she said, calmly.

She read the letter aloud, and as she did, she pointed out—and cackled at—all the typos and misspelled words. Kathy said that my mother should use the dildo on herself now that she didn't have Ron's big cock to fuck her and how my mother was a stupid cunt.

Gaby and I periodically looked at each other and opened our eyes wide in a kind of mock horror. We were loving this turn of events.

When she was finished reading, she put the letter down and said, "Well, this really takes the cake. See kids? I told you she knew. So I'm not crazy after all. She sabotaged me. She *engineered* the entire thing! She destroyed my nose along with that quack Salatin."

And that was it.

She had solved the puzzle of the nose and now she was going to sue The Quack Salatin.

She decided to stop taking the lithium. She didn't need it anymore. She had the lawsuit. And besides, she said, the lithium made her asshole itch.

While Gaby and I waited for our old mother to return—the mother who was not spaced out, the mother with an edge, the mother with a purpose, the mother without an itchy asshole—we hunkered down and disappeared into another episode of *Charles in Charge*.

Chapter 24

The Hour of Regret
and Remorse

N ow that Anthony wants a piece of Gaby's fame, we really have
to get organized. I never should have let Gaby do that movie
for such a paltry amount of money. She's famous now. We'll end up
spending it all on lawyers and fighting that fucking bastard," she
said as we entered the apartment.

It was the summer of '89.

Our old mother was back.

Anthony had taken Gaby to Mississippi to meet his family. She
was terrified before she left. We had to pry her little hands off the
doorframe. We were all crying.

Ron and Kathy were the new enemies, and research on the ill
effects of cortisone was being filed away.

My mother arranged for a friend to hand The Quack Salatin a
subpoena.

The apartment was incredibly empty without Gaby. It tormented me to watch her suffer through the custody battle and go
off into the hands of Anthony, but I had to remind myself that he

wasn't the actual devil as much as our mother believed him to be, and most likely Gaby would be OK.

I would be gone for most of the summer. The Squat's play "*L*" *Train to Eldorado* would be on a European tour. Eva had arranged a small part for me, and I would be flying to Vienna with Rebi and the rest of the troupe in June.

It tormented me even more to imagine abandoning Gaby to the chaos of our mother, to the stress of the movie sets, but I had to keep moving forward and trust that Gaby had the skills to survive without me.

What did I know anyway?

My impending departure was making me nostalgic, and I started riffling through my mother's closet to see if there was anything of hers I wanted to take to Europe.

"You're going to stretch out that dress, honey," she said when I put on the black Betsey Johnson dress she wore all the time when she was pregnant with Gaby. I also loved her fuchsia Ferragamo high heels ("Ferragamos are the only shoes that are narrow enough for my feet"), but her feet were at least two sizes smaller than mine. I took off the dress and as I wandered into the bathroom in my underwear, my mother yelled out: "Oh, God! You walk just like your father! I can't look . . . He sure was great to travel with . . ."

My mother, as usual, was going through papers in the living room. She had the Wite-Out open and the rubber cement at hand.

"Thank God I stopped taking the lithium," she was saying to herself. "They'll use it against me in court. I think it gave me diarrhea too. I never should have gotten that *fucking face-lift*."

"No more coulda, shoulda, woulda," I said firmly.

My mother's big eye was looking at me from the spine of *Superstar*.

I pulled it out along with *The Baby* and lay down on the big bed with the books, staring, for a moment, at Gaby's empty bottom bunk with an aching heart.

I flipped through some pages in *Superstar* until I found a lesbian sex scene.

"Mom," I called out to the living room, "I never knew you liked pussy!"

"It's *FICTION*!" she yelled.

She came into the bedroom and grabbed the book from my hands.

"OK, OK, OK," I said, laughing.

"Disgusting! Oh my God," she said, hiding the book in a drawer.

She lay down next to me. Tupi stood on her hind legs and clawed on her thigh.

"Owww!" she screamed and swatted her away. "Get away from me!"

Tupi jumped on the bed and curled up at her feet.

"It's all made up, honey," she said.

"Sure it is," I said.

She wedged her arm under my shoulders and pulled me in closer.

"I'll be so lonely without you and Gaby," she said.

"Gaby will be home soon," I reassured her. "I, on the other hand, will never return."

"Ha ha," she said.

I let her pull me in closer. I thought, *I should tell her how much I love her,* but we lay there for a while together, and I didn't say anything. I tried to project forward into the future, to imagine coming home to the apartment in my twenties, Gaby as an adult, but nothing came.

Instead, my mind arrived at an amorphous boundary, an inky blob.

At that moment, I had no idea that on a future weekend I will arrive home from Bard College to find both of them covered in plaster dust, chunks of wall in a pile after sledgehammering Sydney's wall down the day she moved out, giving Gaby her own room—and never telling Stanley.

On my mother's desk in the living room and under a pile of family court papers, I will find some mug shots of Gaby. She will have returned from Mississippi with evidence of what, in my mother's opinion, was the most neglectful, inane parental behavior of all time: a sunburn. Anthony will have forgotten to apply sunblock. My mother will take a few Polaroids to use in court.

I will examine the photos: Gaby standing against one of the dirty white stucco walls, naked from the waist up; her hair wild and long, her dark brown eyes downcast; the white outline of her bikini will look ghostly in contrast with the bright red of the burn, her expression deadpan.

"That's all it takes to ruin the skin," my mother will say. "One bad burn. That fucking bastard!"

In the new room we will use the little sink to brush our teeth before bed. In the night I will hear my mother shuffling around in her own bedroom. I will look around the new room Gaby will have made for herself. It will feel like a portal into the unknown, a space that is all hers. It will make me feel better about not living with her. I will be relieved to see her Walkman, her posters, her Rollerblades. I will look out the window and watch a plane cutting a path through the stars, and I will remember my mother trying to explain the concept of infinity to me.

My mother and Gaby will move out of the apartment while I am in Budapest with Rebi.

My mother will forever lament the loss of the apartment, frequently saying, "I can't believe I let Stanley kick us out of that apartment. It had such great light!"

And the word *light*—as it always has been—will be infused with a deeper meaning, as though the elusive presence of perfect light signifies an unattainable material and spiritual success.

In the first weeks of college I will wake up at dawn, half asleep, and be temporarily convinced that I have to make contact with my mother in order to make sense of things, in order to remember who I am; it will seem eons since we last saw each other; and this illusion of lost time will terrify me.

But after a minute I will come to my senses and be fine.

My mother will be writing her own "Spiritual Memoirs."

Gaby will make more movies, and earn more money, and they will move to a white tiled ranch house, with a pool, in the Valley. They will buy a white shabby chic down-filled couch.

When Gaby is twelve, she will pluck her bushy eyebrows into tidy thin arches. Mom will make a serial-killer-like collage of bushy eyebrows, roughly cut from faces in magazines, and tape it to her bedroom door. She will tape a note next to one set of eyebrows that says *BROOKE SHIELDS* written in red capital letters with arrows pointing to them.

After Gaby leaves home at sixteen to live, for a while, with Michel and Cindy in NYC, Mom will begin a kind of nomadic journey, with extended summer visits to the River. During those visits she will take over the house after the family leaves, finally the lord of the manor, freely spreading coffee-filter socks around the kitchen and leaving just before things freeze over.

Every few years she will either get fed up with her location or get evicted from where she has settled.

On September 11, 2001, a U-Haul will be barreling down the

Thruway from Syracuse with all her furniture, files, archives, and clothes; barreling toward a storage unit near my little house in Hudson, where I will be living with Nick. It will be a strange coincidence that I will have scheduled the U-Haul for that morning. When the planes hit the towers, she will call and say, "Abort the mission! Stay inside! I'm calling the movers and telling them to turn around! The terrorists are going to hit the Thruway, I just know it! All my files will be destroyed!"

Gaby will have slept at our house the night before, with a few friends, and we will all meet the U-Haul, red-eyed from crying over the burning towers on TV.

We will all stand in a line from the inside of the U-Haul to the entrance of the storage unit. We will pass each other boxes. We will pause at times and look into the haphazardly packed boxes, some open.

We will see a single shoe and a tub of gesso in one box.

We will see her collection of books about Warhol, a book about lizard-like aliens in human form running the world (nonfiction), and books about string theory.

I will pass the box that holds the copies of her own books, and her big eye will stare at me again from the spine of one. I'll take that book.

We will pass files down the line, and we will read the labels aloud before we stuff them back into the filing cabinet inside the storage unit: Aliens, Aids, Atrophied Skin, Baby M, Bad Fathers, Black Mold, Botched Plastic Surgery, Child Pornography, Cortisone, Radiation, Tupamaros.

My mother will call again and say, "Take the couch, honey. Who knows if I'll ever have my own house again? I'll probably be penniless and homeless. You'll abandon me and send me to a nursing home, I know it. But take the couch, really. The covers are *all re-movable*. They can all be washed. You can use bleach. I even put them in the dryer. There are a couple of stains. There's one stain where Tupi bled on . . ."

I will not know that there will be lifelong consequences from taking the couch; that from then on my mother will ask about the couch like it was another grandchild; that when she gets upset, she will say, "And now I'm homeless and penniless, and you and Gaby and your father all have your own houses, and now you have my couch"; and when she visits, she will tell us to keep our dirty feet off the couch, and she will ask how the new stains got there, and she will tell my friends not to eat while they are sitting on the couch, and if anyone lets their dogs on the couch, she will get really mad and say: "I'm taking my fucking couch back!"

Her dogs will have multiplied. She will have bred them. They will be allowed on the couch.

According to her, Gaby will have abandoned the dogs to her, starting with that dog her asshole father gave her.

Gaby's father will periodically try to connect with her; Gaby will periodically try to connect with him. Her father will die.

Joe will die, and Fred Beverly too, both from cancer.

Ron will live, and so will Bill Eggleston. In fact, on a cross-country drive, Nick and I will stop in Memphis to see Bill, but when we arrive, Rowzah will tell us he's "not in a state" to come down the stairs.

Bob Fulton will die from crashing his own plane. I will meet Marybeth and some of my cousins at the cow pasture where Bob's plane went down. We will help the farmer recover as many pieces of the plane as we can so that the cows don't choke. I will find pieces of Bob too, wedged into tufts of grass and dirt—a slice of scalp with a sprout of gray hair, and a single pearl key—and I will think, *God how I hated it when we had to listen to him play the sax.*

The dogs will live for a while as my mother's cohorts, her minions, her white devils. She will have a cauldron going on the stove at all times—a thick cast-iron pot of coagulating rice and bones for the dogs surrounded by old socks draped over the edges of countertops, stiff and yellowed from the dried coffee inside them.

The dogs will follow her everywhere. They will bite kids and bleed on the couch. There will be a blood trail through whatever space she is in and we will wonder aloud who got injured, and she will say, "Shit, Tupi got her period again." They will sidle up next to her and claw her leg for attention, and we will startle when she screams: "Oooh! I can't stand it anymore! Get away from me!"

I will call her to see how she is doing, and the dogs will always be somewhere high up on the litany of complaints. "I think it's the air here in Santa Monica. The Santa Ana wind is driving me crazy. I mean if I'm painting at Point Dume, I'm fine, but I need an air purifier. Well, I'm penniless, so ha! Wouldn't you know, everyone owns a house but me. Your father. You. Gaby. Gaby just sent me $1,000, but that's gone already. I mean I just don't have time to deal with these dogs. I'm just exhausted, Alex, I have no help, I have to walk the dogs, *Gaby's* dogs—I'm going to have to send them back to her, or else I'll have to put them down . . . poor dogs, here Runtie, here's the lamb chop; oh, you want more? They're Gaby's dogs, you know. She begged for a dog . . ."

"Mom, she was seven," I will say.

"In third world countries the whole family lives together, they help each other! This is the only country . . . Oh, never mind! You girls don't give a shit! Wait until I'm dead! Wait until you have kids of your own! Just you wait!" she will say.

Tupi will get hit by a car in front of her and die. She will be so upset she will get transient global amnesia, probably brought on by some mystery migraine pills her neighbor gave her. We won't know this when she calls us over and over again to describe the violent death, each time, as though she hadn't just told us a minute before.

During one of the calls, I will have her write down how the dog died so that the next time she calls, she will be able to go to her kitchen table and read the story of the dog's death in her own hand-writing. I will be hoping that will snap her out of it.

When she calls again, I will say, "Mom, read me the letter on your kitchen table."

"OK," she will say. "Here it is: 'I went out to get the groceries from the car, Tupi ran after me and got hit by a van as she tried . . .'" And at that point she will interrupt herself and wail, "Oh my God, is she OK?!" Then we will have to break the news again, and she will start sobbing as though it were the very first she had heard of it.

I will be temporarily certain, resolved even, that it is the end for her.

I will fantasize about dictating a new letter—like I did with the dog death story—that she will write herself and read back to me. It will say: "I was a high-maintenance mother, I screamed all the time, I'm sorry I forced you to talk to your father about his drug addiction, I had no boundaries . . ."

But I will never get the note right in my head; I will never be able to get to the essence of what I want her to confess to me.

Now

She is examining the shabby chic couch like an English butler doing a white-glove test, disdainfully picking up the corner of the fraying Indian bedspread that we use to cover up the rips and stains on the white upholstery underneath.

How long has she been with us now?

We celebrated the new year, this I know, but she stayed home in bed.

Don't ask about the departure date, I remind myself.

But she reserved a flight, this I know. This feeds me. This brings me slowly back to the surface.

Now she lays herself out on the surprisingly still fluffy down cushions.

"They don't make couches like this anymore," she says.

"It's true," I say, sitting down next to her.

"You need to get it reupholstered. You know these slipcovers come right off and you can put them right in the washing machine."

"No! They come off?!"

"You're kidding, I know."

I should tell her I love her before she leaves.

Instead, I'm silent.

"Sorry, honey," she says. "I know I'm a burden. It's just such hell getting old."

———

I've decided to try to cuddle with her on this last night before she leaves. I get in the single bed and slide my arm under her shoulders.

It's similar to cuddling a body going through puberty.

It feels like the distance between us can't be physically spanned.

They say the cosmos is a hunk of Swiss cheese, and each hole is its own universe and the cheese in between is dark energy expanding at a rate that makes it impossible to traverse the cheese and get to the next universe. And in the holes there are bound to be replicas of you and me because there is a finite amount of matter in an infinite amount of space.

It's three thirty a.m., when I know nothing and fear the worst.

Just an hour or so after both of my kids were born I looked into their eyes and imagined them dying. I imagined their translucent lips and pin-prick nostrils taking their final breath.

How did I end up here?

Who are these bodies in this house?

Who is this hunk of flesh next to me, breathing?

Lui needs me. Check on her now! No, I'm being crazy. Or am I? She's sleeping in the bedroom right down the hall. Or is she? If I go now, I could stop her just in time . . .

I remain still, looking out the window at the foot of our bed, watching the black branches.

Go see if she's in bed.

I should have lit candles on the dinner table every night, I think, like Gaby does. They say dinnertime makes or breaks a family.

Why did we scrunch ourselves into that too small kitchen table for so long?

I drank too much while I cooked.

I was a crabby, cunty martyr.

Why did I ridicule the preciousness of the Waldorf parents and the earnestness of the Quakers?

If I had forced the children to set the table and light beeswax candles in simple Shaker candleholders, would Lui still be bathed in the evil blue light, watching movies on her laptop at this hour?

The blue light!

If I had not ridiculed the parents who made their children say please and thank you—would Miko accept less screen time?

I tried not to tell the kids about all my feelings all the time, but what did I do instead? Did I have any methodology at all?

If I go now, I could stop her just in time . . .

Once, at three thirty, I heeded the call and slipped out of bed to go check on her. She was gone.

Gone!

Her bed was actually empty.

Now I throw myself out of bed to go check on her.

Her body is there, breathing, her face glowing blue.

I close the laptop.

I smell her breath.

Cigarettes.

I go back to bed and have a nightmare. These days nightmares are populated by the most frightening creatures of all: teenagers.

In the nightmare Lui is walking down the hall trying to leave the house. I get up and follow her. She has her back to me, her shoulders exposed in her white tank top.

Lui, I say, trying to catch up to her as I follow her down the stairs.

She doesn't answer, doesn't turn to look at me.

Lui!

She intends to escape.

I scream her name again.

She turns around.

It's not her—it's a teenage boy!

He leads me through the open doors of the screen porch and locks me in and sits on my chest, smothering me.

He's the Night Hag now.

More teens appear, and they trash the porch. They throw Miko's toys into the air like confetti, blasting songs about pussy licking and dick sucking, chucking large pieces of furniture through the screens.

I try to scream at them to get out, but they can't hear me because the Night Hag has devoured my voice.

I slip out of bed again to go stand in the hall and listen for breathing.

I hear my mother lightly snoring.

I see Lui's body under the blankets.

Tomorrow I'll send my mother home to settle back into her own mess.

I climb back into bed with Nick and Miko. Miko throws a leg over my waist, attaches to me like a sea urchin, kissing me, caressing my face with his hot little hands.

I inhale his exhale, our mouths close together.

He's not afraid of my breath yet.

"Do you love me more than you love yourself?" he asks me.

The time has come.

We are packing Viva's stuff into the car so I can drive her to the airport.

"You better lose some weight, Nick," she says, hugging him. "Any day you could drop dead from that belly fat."

"Thanks, Viva, love you," he says.

The kids offer their goodbyes, hug and kiss her.

"This may be the last time you'll ever see me," she tells them.

While I'm driving, I try to think of things to say.

Nothing comes.

I put my hand on her leg.

"We will miss you," I say.

We are at the airport.

"Well, that's it! You'll most likely never see me again. This was my last trip! I'm just too old. This trip almost killed me," she says.

"You say that every time," I say. "Remember, I even made some videos called 'Viva's last so and so . . .' That was ten years ago."

"Well, this really is the last time I'll travel."

I have to hunch over a bit to hug her. I jokingly bury my face in her neck and tickle her with my chin and make baby sounds. Her skin is surprisingly sweet smelling, her coarse hair falls over my eyes.

Suddenly I feel the prickle of tears.

This is unexpected.

She notices and hugs me closer.

OK, I'm crying in front of her, I think. *No big deal.*

I have not let myself cry in front of her for a long, long time. Maybe decades.

Whenever Gaby and I see her off at the airport together, the moment she is out of sight, we walk away and give each other a look. When I have tried to describe this look to friends, they say: "You mean because you're so sad to see her leave?"

No.

The look is relief. Then guilt and terror. Relief to be rid of her. Guilt for having been such rancid cunts. And terror that it could, actually, turn out to be her last visit, and if so, we failed.

I continue to hug her and cry, distancing myself from the action, telling myself with a sarcastic snort that this is good exposure therapy.

Things will be easier between us from here on out, I think to myself.

My face is still nuzzled in her neck, and I'm still crying. I'm crying because I can't forgive. I'm crying from the relief of finally getting her out of my house. Crying because we can't tell our story together and crying because we can't seem to agree on it.

My mother, on the other hand, thinks I'm crying about something else.

She abruptly pulls away and begins to vigorously rub my chest.

"Honey!" she gasps. She looks me in the eyes. "I was *just* kiiiiidding! I promise I won't die!"

She abruptly pulls me back into the hug.

"I *promise*!" she reiterates.

After a beat she grasps my shoulders and pushes me away *again* to do more of the vigorous chest-rubbing thing.

"I forgive you," she says solemnly.

She pulls me back into the hug again.

"Don't worry!" she reassures me, squeezing me tight. "I forgive you, I forgive you, sweetie . . . I forgive you . . ."

My breath quiets. I write Gaby a text in my head: *Guess what? Mom just forgave ME, ha ha, ha ha, ha ha!*

I stay nestled in her neck, still, my lips touching her pulse; it's telling me something, something in Morse code; I try to decipher the gentle thuds. They speak to me of potential.

Or no!

What is it then?

Portents! They speak to me of plagues! They speak to me of con-
spiracies and deeper rifts to come!

I quickly pull away.

She disappears into the plane, taking her pulse with her. I can still
feel it speaking to me as the plane gets smaller and smaller in the sky.

Acknowledgments

When Meg Leder—my beloved editor to whom I offer my first out-pouring of gratitude—finished reading the first draft of this book, she said something like, "You know, Alex, I just read that the Natural History Museum only displays about three percent of their entire collection . . ."

Because I've been writing versions of this story for over twenty-five years, and each draft has had an imaginary acknowledgments page, the list of people I'm indebted to has grown exponentially. I'll try to be brief, Meg, but it's going to be hard.

I'm particularly indebted to two women, both incredible writers, who used copious amounts of their precious time to help me with a much older version of this book: Elizabeth Frank and Jo Ann Beard. Liz was one of my professors at Bard College, and after I graduated, she kindly offered to edit the original—fictional—version of this story, and then she kindly gave it to her agent, who suggested it should be nonfiction. Sometime after that I landed in the tender arms of Jo Ann, who miraculously agreed to help me turn it into a memoir. Thank you both a million times!

Long story short, I put the book into a bottom drawer for about a decade.

Then Katherine Rosman (thank you!) said something that made me pull it out of the drawer.

Elisa Albert, thank you for your wickedly funny voice in my ear, for your willingness to give me frank advice/reads at any hour, and for letting me write to Sarah Bowlin. And thank you, Sarah Bowlin, for that indispensable time—your input, advice, and encouragement ushered me forward.

Sam, I'm so grateful you mentioned my name at that party.

Jynne Martin? Jynne Martin? Jynne Martin? Even though you never showed up to my yoga class, and I sheepishly called out your name before I began to teach to see if you were there because I wanted to kiss your ass, I owe the start of this process to you. Thank you for helping me home in on the story I wanted to tell, and for introducing me to Marya.

Marya Spence! Get out of here, you are too good to be true. Marry me? Even though I'm already married to Nick? If you are reading this, it means Armageddon didn't happen before this book was published as I had predicted. You were right. But I do need to wear a diaper now.

Catherine Cacki Martin and Catriona Briger, thank you for enthusiastically reading anything and everything I threw at you— from proposal to final draft—and then quickly offering the most thoughtful, efficient, and intelligent feedback despite being overworked and underfed yourselves.

Tara Culp, thank you for giving me such a beautiful little room with a view and for making my fantasy come true by delivering food to my door so I could pretend I was at MacDowell.

Patsy Cummings, I am so lucky you and Viva were (and still are!) the best of friends and that you let us share the beautiful life you and Joe created in Zihua.

Claire Dederer, thank you for getting on the phone with me at the very moment I needed your advice.

Thank you, Molly Ringwald and Parker Posey, for reading the very long proposal and offering your flattery and kind blurbs.

Marianne Vitale! A million thanks and more for your bottomless pit of generosity.

Jane Lancellotti, thank you for your thorough reads and hearty laughs.

Thank you: Layla Childs, Alisoun Meehan, Chris Meehan, Jesse James, Kostas Anagnopoulos, Eszter Balint, Megan Kane, Nikki Vilella, Lauren Haythe, Abby Klein, Momlandia, Book Club Bitches, Kula Yoga, Nicole Meadors, Rachel Comey, Todd Thomas, the Stone family, Annie Leibovitz, Joy Harris, Erika Storella, and Shubhraj.

Thank you, Rebecca Major, for being the best friend a girl could have, and Eva Buchmuller, for taking me in and feeding me so well, and the Squat Theatre.

Thank you again, Meg Leder, for organizing my mind, and thank you Viking team: Tricia Conley, Linda Friedner, Sharon Gonzalez, Annika Karody, Anna Scheithauer, Andrea Schulz, Brian Tart, and Colin Webber.

Thanks to all my Hoffmann aunts and uncles, all my cousins (I'm sorry, you are just too many to name, Meg will kill me!), Sue Dapkins, Chris Dapkins, sister Val Nehez, brother Anthony Tyler, nieces LillyBelle and Hazel, Father Nick Nehez Sr., and deep gratitude to the world's greatest mother-in-law/editor, Carole Nehez.

Cindy, thank you for being my other mother and for sticking with us through thick and thin. I could not have written this book without you.

Dad, thank you for being so cool and supportive about everything I wrote and always sending me whatever material I needed right away.

Gaby, your love and support have bolstered me through this process. Thank you.

Lui, thank you for your sweet support, unconditional acceptance, and stellar wit, for your beauty inside and out, and for keeping me from getting canceled.

Miko, thank you for being the most loving, fun, and funny kid to live with, and for helping me choose the book jacket.

Nick, thank you for a lifetime of support and laughter. Thanks for that very important final read, for your thorough editing notes, for your patience with my technological idiocy, and for feeding me the best one-liners.

I could go on, but I won't.